DEDICATION

In my works of fiction, I typically thank those who have stood by me and supported me during the creative process. In this case, I must thank those who stood by me while I spent more than a week in the hospital undergoing surgery and then through months of recovery as I regained my strength.

To all of you who sent me cards or notes, texts or calls, thank you. It was nearly overwhelming at times, but it was deeply appreciated none-the-less. So many friends stopped by or offered to help, or fixed a meal to take the pressure off of my wife Beverly. I can never repay that, but I will try.

To my family, I am sorry to put you through this. I wish I had recognized, or admitted, the signs and symptoms earlier and never scared you at all. Regardless, you stood by me when I was moody or in pain and I love you. This book is for you all; my way of saying thank you.

Heart Survivor:

Recovery After Heart Surgery

ERIC DOUGLAS

ISBN-10: 1542439345
ISBN-13: 978-1542439343

Table of Contents

Foreword

At the age of 48 years, Eric Douglas who is an EMT, CPR instructor, and author of untold articles on scuba diving safety, underwent five vessel coronary artery bypass surgery – an operation most people feel is reserved for the elderly. Like most young people with coronary artery disease, he felt his symptoms had to be from something else. He couldn't possibly have coronary artery disease. He was too young. As an interventional cardiologist, I have seen far too many patients over the years who have had to deal with the same reality.

Eric has spent his career as a journalist making scuba diving safer for millions of divers worldwide while also penning multiple novels and short stories that often have an element of scuba diving. I have known him through our joint work with the Divers Alert Network (DAN) for whom I am a cardiology consultant. His current book, Heart Survivor, is a wonderful blend of the science and statistics of coronary artery disease with personal insights from his own journey as well as the journey of others coping with coronary artery disease.

Unlike many books on the subject aimed at the general population, Heart Survivor gives the reader a patient's perspective as Eric was unexpectedly thrust into a medical system of tests, procedures, surgeries, and rehabilitation along with all of the emotional baggage that brings. Being an accomplished author with medical knowledge makes this a very enjoyable read. In the book, Eric explains his most intimate thoughts and feelings at each point along the way – the diagnosis, the surgery, cardiac rehabilitation, and beyond – in a manner that commands the attention of the reader. His use of responses from many other survivors regarding their own personal experiences and insights with cardiac disease gives the book an additional personal aspect to interest the reader.

This is a book I will recommend highly to all of my coronary artery disease patients so they can see what lies ahead of them from the perspectives of others who are farther along on their own road to recovery.

Douglas Ebersole, MD
Interventional Cardiologist, Watson Clinic LLP
Cardiology Consultant, Divers Alert Network

Chapter 1: Introduction

Charleston Gazette-Mail

Don't make the same mistake I did

By Eric Douglas

February 3, 2016

Entering the hospital, I passed a friend from church who was going home.

The first thing she told me was how much she enjoyed these columns. And then she asked why I was at the hospital. I hadn't had a chance to tell my family, primarily my daughters, at that point, so I evaded the question as well as I could.

Recently, something happened in my life that has changed my perspective on, well, just about everything. I went to see a cardiologist because I was experiencing some chest discomfort. (I was sure it was just heartburn. I was way too young to have heart problems.)

By the end of the day, I had been admitted to the hospital and was waiting on a heart catheterization and probable stent. After the heart cath, they determined there were blockages and I was going to have to have bypass surgery.

There are so many clichés about events like this. Every one of them makes the writer in me flinch, so I will do my best to avoid them. Still, when you fail a stress test (I told the doctor I've always been good at taking tests...), it is definitely a wake-up call. While I don't plan to completely shift the focus of this column to talking about my heart, I imagine it will come up regularly in the next few months as I work through cardiac rehab and improve my overall health. If you can learn something while I learn it, we both benefit.

For now, I will say, don't think you are "too young" or "it can't happen to me, I have no family history." I am 48 and have no family history of heart disease, either. But I have severe coronary artery blockages and have heard it said several times already that I'm lucky it just didn't kill me.

Pay attention to the warning signs: Chest pain and discomfort. Shortness of breath, especially on exertion. Pain in the chest after exertion. Decreased ability to exercise or do physical work. I had all of those. In hindsight, I realize I've been denying them for several months now.

In a previous life, my job was creating CPR-related training programs and teaching people to be instructors and instructor trainers in CPR. I've held the rating of "Master" trainer.

I still denied what was going on and justified it away, even though I knew the symptoms backward and forward.

Don't make the same mistake I did. You might not be as lucky.

#

What you just read was a column I wrote for my local newspaper while I was in the hospital waiting for open-heart surgery. I've 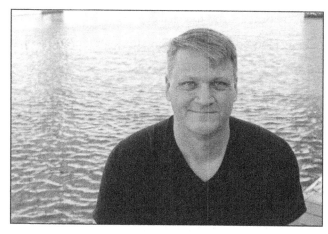 included several columns I wrote about my recovery process in this book.

I am a heart survivor. Until about a year ago, I wouldn't have even known what that meant. I had a heart attack that I denied, writing it off as heartburn even though I should know better. When I finally went to the cardiologist, I was swept away down a river of doctors, surgery and rehabilitation, often feeling out of control and just along for the ride. I ended up having open-heart surgery. I will never forget one of the nurses asking me if I was in the hospital for a "cabbage." I had no idea what she meant. She was using medical slang for CABG: coronary artery bypass graft. I had five of them.

If you are reading this I assume you are a heart or stroke survivor or know someone who is. I have been public about the rehab and recovery process because I wanted to inspire my friends who might not be in the best of shape and/or had risk factors to talk to their doctors and make changes in their lives. I also wanted to help others going through the same process to understand what they would be facing. A close friend had the same surgery about six months after mine. He told me he felt prepared for the process after following me.

This book is not about me telling you how easy it was for me. Or how hard it was, for that matter. This book is simply my thoughts on the recovery process and the challenges I faced. I doubt any of mine were unique. Honestly, I think I came through it pretty well, but I don't think I am special because of it.

In this book, you will find three things:

First, you will see a series of newspaper columns I wrote about the process. The first one was written before my surgery and published the day I was released from the hospital. I've inserted them at appropriate times throughout the book. They may be a little redundant, but I think that's okay. Some of the points probably bear repeating.

Second, you will read my memories of the process in more detail than I could address in those weekly columns.

Third, you'll see the thoughts and recollections of a group of other heart and stroke survivors. I set up a survey on my website and asked survivors what helped them through their recoveries. Where appropriate, I followed up with them to get an idea what worked and what didn't. I think you will find some of their stories enlightening.

There are any number of nicknames for those of us who have had open-heart surgery. Members of the Zipper Club and Team Second Chance are a couple that I like to use. Ultimately, the only label that matters is survivor.

Statistics

More than 100 heart and stroke survivors responded to my survey. It wasn't perfect and it doesn't qualify as being "scientific" for several reasons, but the results are interesting anyway. I think they are a representative sample of survivors and our experiences.

Some people came through the process with little or no problem, while others are still struggling years after their initial cardiac event. If anyone tells you they have a silver bullet or a trick that will make all your problems go away, they are lying to you. If you are a heart or stroke survivor, your body has endured a tremendous insult. It takes time and determination to make a recovery. For some people, you may never regain full strength or complicating medical factors may hold you back. Those stories are all represented in the survey respondents.

The survey included both Yes or No questions and opportunities for short answers. I wanted to be able to develop an overall picture on who the average respondent to the survey was before getting off into the individual stories. The rest of this section is about the who, using averages and statistics gained from the survey questions.

As I said, this isn't a scientific survey. First, the sample size isn't large enough to truly represent heart and stroke survivors. Second, these people chose to answer the survey, rather than being a blind or random polling of heart and stroke survivors. We can't really take these numbers and apply them to the population. Rather, this will give you an idea of who the people were as you read through their anecdotes and comments throughout the rest of the text.

Gender and Age

Too often we think of heart disease as being a male problem, but 51 percent of the respondents to the survey were women. We also assume that it is a problem for older people. Respondents to the survey ranged in age from 21- to 79-years-of-age. The average age of all respondents was 53.6 years.

Gender

Male   49%

Female   51%

Average age by Gender

Men   56

Women   51

Diagnosis

Often, we imagine that people have a heart attack and are rushed to the hospital where they are diagnosed with blockages and have surgery or receive stents or other medical interventions. Sixty nine percent of the respondents to the survey did fall into that category, but another 31 percent, myself included, received the diagnosis without an "event". They weren't feeling well and went to their doctor, only to find out that they had blockages. A fair number of those likely had events that they overlooked, ignored, or denied only to find out later that the doctor found evidence of a previous stroke or heart attack. That was how it happened for me.

Diagnosis without event   31%

Diagnosis after stroke or heart attack   69%

Procedure

Nearly all the respondents were heart survivors and most of them endured cardiac bypass surgery.

Bypass: 54.5%

Stents: 40%

Other   5.5%

Did you have a goal when you began your recovery?

Having a goal is an important part of recovery. I believe it has to be something more concrete than "get in better shape" or "lose some weight." A goal must be measurable. You have to have a finish line to cross or how would you know if you achieved it? I will discuss this more later.

Yes   77%

No   23%

Formal Rehab Program

Cardiac rehabilitation programs help survivors get back on their feet and learn to exercise under the watchful eye of exercise physiologists and nurses. I was surprised that only about two-thirds of the respondents completed a formal rehab program. Later, you'll read the whys of this and what the ones who did gained from the program.

No formal rehab   35%

Rehab   65%

Recovery Time

In the hospital I began telling myself that this recovery process was going to take some time. I set myself a goal that I hoped to reach six months after being released, but I knew at the time it was optimistic. I asked the respondents how long their recovery took. These are the percentages from those who felt they had recovered as much as they were going to following surgery.

3-4 months   20%

| 6-9 months | 20% |
| 12+ | 60% |

Changes

For most people, it is important to make changes to diet and exercise to be able to complete your recovery. Some of the respondents may have already had an exercise program, or been eating a healthy diet so they only needed to work on one aspect for their personal recovery. Most of us, though, needed to work on everything.

Diet	21%
Exercise	9%
Both diet and exercise	69%

Strength after recovery

One interesting series of responses came from the question about the perceived strength after recovery. A surprising amount of people didn't feel as if they were stronger than before.

Not as strong	60%
As strong as before	18%
Stronger than before	21%

When I first started looking at the numbers, I imagined the people who didn't feel as strong were probably older. That wasn't the case. (These percentages are slightly different, because not all respondents answered both the age and the strength questions.)

Strength when adjusted for age		Av Age
Not as strong	59.6%	53.7
As strong as before	17%	54.8
Stronger than before	23%	52.4

I am a firm believer in cardiac rehab, but it doesn't seem to have a direct correlation to how people feel once they are done.

Respondents who did not complete formal rehab

Not as strong as before	57%
As strong as	20%
Stronger than	22%

Respondents who completed a rehab program

Not as strong as before	61%
As strong as	16%
Stronger than	22%

My guess is some of these numbers surprised you. You may have thought you were the "only one" or "too young." I know I did when I began my recovery. Numbers, however, cannot tell the human story. They just set the stage. Throughout the rest of this book, you will read actual survivor stories. Some people came through the process nearly unscathed. Others are still struggling with their recovery for any number of reasons.

Chapter 2: Denial

Charleston Gazette-Mail

No more broken hearts at Valentine's Day

By Eric Douglas

February 11, 2016

Over the last few months, I've noticed a few odd things about the way I've been feeling.

In fact, now that I think about it, those odd feelings go all the way back to last summer. I remember getting winded mowing the grass and feeling embarrassed. I told myself that I must've let myself get in terrible shape. I hoped none of my neighbors saw me bending over, still holding onto the lawnmower, to catch my breath. You probably read about this in my column last week.

There are other instances from the last few months, but you get the idea. The last few weeks, before my doctor's appointment, one of my greatest concerns was to not mess up the holidays while rationalizing that what I was feeling couldn't be related to my heart.

In all, the surgeon performed five bypasses on my heart

a couple weeks ago. And then I spent five more nights in the hospital beginning the recovery process. As my wife and I have discussed several times already, the looming lifestyle changes and eating habits are a marathon, not a sprint.

Since I announced through social media that I was having heart surgery, an incredible number of my friends have told me their personal stories. One friend jokingly admitted me into the "broken hearts club." My younger daughter told me that some people celebrate a situation like this by considering the day after surgery as their new birthday.

With this weekend's Valentine holiday fast approaching, the odds are good that I won't make it to the store to get my wife a gift. I now realize that worrying about not messing up the holidays would just have made the rest of them worse if I had keeled over in the snow.

So, my Valentine gift this year is a bit indirect. It's about me, but it's for them. I promise to take better care of my own heart so there will be many more valentines in the future. Birthdays, too. And no more broken hearts.

My guess is your loved ones will appreciate that as much as a box of chocolates. (But you do have to put in the work, too.)

Who am I

At this point, I should probably explain a bit more about my background so you understand where I am coming from. My name is Eric Douglas and I am a heart survivor. I like that phrase, but I also find it a little odd. I survived a heart attack and quintuple bypass surgery. I've survived cardiac rehab and have worked my tail off to get my life back.

My story is important because it's unusual and it's not. I'm 49 years old

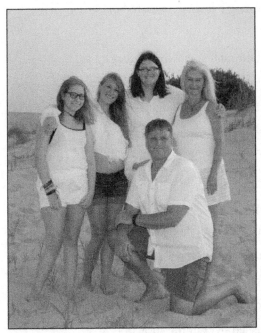

and have no family history of heart disease. I am not a super athlete, but I have always been active. I'm a scuba diver and have made a living for the last 20 years or so traveling the world teaching about scuba diving and dive safety. I'm also a son, a husband and a father.

One of the keys to this story, though, is that I am a full-time writer. I work from home and go to work every day with my computer. I tell stories for a living. What I've gone through, and what I'm writing about now, is the most important story I will ever tell as far as I'm concerned.

To back up a bit, I was born in the summer of 1967 in Charleston, West Virginia. I grew up what I would call lower middle class. I didn't have everything, but I don't remember wanting for a whole lot either. My brother and I have talked about it many times that we thought we had a good childhood. We played outside, rode horses, swam and did all the things kids growing up in the 70s did. I remember getting a home weight set at 11 or 12 years old. My brother and I would work out and that expanded into high school and college. In my 20s, I could bench press 365 pounds and squat and deadlift more than 400 pounds each.

Of course, growing up in Appalachia in the 70s and early 80s came with lots of casseroles and fried food. I spent a lot of time in my 20s in the gym, but I also spent a lot of time at the bar, consuming loads of empty calories. Still, I could balance it all out. I never had six-pack abs, but I carried my body well.

I bring all of that up simply to suggest that while I was active and relatively fit in my youth, my guess is my heart disease began back then.

I've been fortunate to tell stories my entire professional life. My degree is in journalism from Marshall University. I've worked in newspapers. I've written for magazines. I've produced photographic and audio documentaries. I've even had a collection of my photographs exhibited in Russia, France and the United States.

Right out of college, I looked at my minimal resume and decided I needed to add something to it that would make me stand out. I decided to learn to scuba dive. That decision gave me the opportunity to move from West Virginia to California to North Carolina. It also took me all over the world, visiting every continent except for Antarctica. The experience and adventure of diving is probably what makes my story interesting.

I said many of the seeds of my heart disease were likely sown in my childhood or youth. My recent history is just as important, however. In the last eight years, I've gotten a divorce, lost my job, moved a couple times and remarried. My stress levels have seen better days. On top of that, working for myself, sometimes wondering how I am going to pay my bills, has kept things tense.

Especially in the last few years I have felt guilty about getting up from my computer and exercising. That was time I felt I should be spending working at my desk. My health took a back seat to the stresses and pressures of daily life.

As I said, my story is different in some ways, but I think it is also extremely typical, too. I've dealt with life stresses. I didn't always eat well or take the best care of myself. Most importantly, I didn't see it coming when the diagnosis came out of left field.

Why I should have known better

In 1998 I moved to California to work in the recreational scuba diving industry. I was working for the Professional Association of Diving Instructors (PADI) and having the time of my life. Every conversation around the water cooler had to do with scuba diving. PADI is the world's largest scuba training agency and we had offices and affiliates all over the world. I was already a diver and a divemaster when I went to work there, but I was hired as a writer. I worked on the quarterly magazine we published as well as on new course development.

Browsing a dive magazine in the office one day, I read about the role of the diver medic in the diving community and set out to earn the certification for myself. My first step was to complete an Emergency Medical Technician (EMT) course at a local community college. I often tell people that I took my first cardiopulmonary resuscitation (CPR) course when I was nine-years-old. I became a CPR instructor in 1999 shortly after becoming a dive instructor, but this was my first real taste of emergency medicine. While the role of the EMT is limited, I absorbed a lot of theory about human physiology and how to provide care in an emergency.

From there, I took a course at the local hyperbaric chamber on how to provide emergency care for injured divers. It was there that I first performed CPR on a real patient. That was an experience I won't ever forget, but the details aren't important. Suffice it to say that the patient did not recover.

That all led me to my next position at Divers Alert Network (DAN). I spent nearly 12 years there running the training department. My job involved developing first aid and CPR courses specific to the diving world. I wrote the organization's first AED training course and then went on to develop a series of CPR courses for the lay provider and for the professional rescuer, writing the manuals and the video scripts. I also organized a course to teach others to be diver medics.

Every five years, I read the latest Emergency Cardiac Care guidelines from the American Heart Association and the International Liaison Committee on Resuscitation.[1] I revised our training programs and demonstrated CPR all over the world. I issued more than 1000 certifications to people who wanted to be CPR Instructors and Instructor Trainers.

Literally every week I discussed CPR, first aid and the issues of the body, health and resuscitation. I know the signs and symptoms of a heart attack and sudden cardiac arrest as well as anyone. I've written the line that Denial is a sign of a heart attack dozens of times.

With all that information, why didn't I recognize Denial in my own situation?

I denied the possibility that I was having a heart-related problem. I ignored it, or justified it away. Most importantly, I didn't tell anyone how I was feeling. I didn't want to alarm my loved ones. And then came my actual diagnosis.

Chapter 3: Diagnosis

My diagnosis

I hadn't been feeling quite right for a few months. I lacked energy and didn't feel like exercising. I was also struggling with heartburn. I would treat it with over-the-counter medications. Sometimes they would work and sometimes they wouldn't.

Finally, I called my family doctor and made an appointment. In passing I mentioned some substernal burning, a burning feeling in my chest. He performed an EKG, but didn't see much that gave him pause. Still, he said, let's schedule a stress test to rule out any problems. After that, he told me, we'll probably do an endoscopy to check for an ulcer or some other stomach problem.

He referred me to a cardiologist he thought highly of and I waited for them to schedule an appointment. It just so happened that when I got the letter from the cardiologist's office, I was going to be out of town the day they had penciled me in. I called them and said I would call them back and reschedule the appointment later. After all, it couldn't be a problem with my heart. This wasn't an emergency so I wasn't in a rush.

When I got back from my trip, it was a couple weeks before Thanksgiving and then Christmas was right around the corner. I put off and postponed calling the doctor again and again. The heartburn came back from time to time, even making it nearly impossible for me to exercise on my home treadmill.

One evening, a week or so before Christmas, in an abnormally warm December, I was out on my friend's boat for a lighted boat parade. I ate some party food and had a couple mixed drinks. That evening when I got home, when I got to the top of the stairs in my house, I got hit with an overwhelming wave of nausea. I had to squat down on the floor for fear of passing out. I broke out into a sweat. It took me about a half an hour to get things back under control. That was the worst the heartburn had ever been. I took some more antacids and went to bed.

While I was still convinced I had severe heartburn, I decided to restart taking the baby aspirin my family doctor had recommended a few months before when I first saw him. I resolved that as soon as Christmas was over, I would call the cardiologist and make an appointment so I could get that out of the way and then figure out what was causing my heartburn. Since it wasn't an emergency, the cardiologist scheduled me for an appointment at the end of January.

My stress test was scheduled for Monday, January 25. On January 22, a massive snow storm hit the area, dropping 18 inches of a dry, light snow. I shoveled snow on Friday and Saturday. Sunday, the sun finally came out and started melting things a bit. I

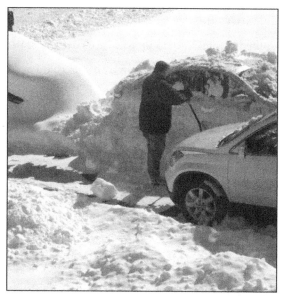

shoveled snow again to clear my car out so I could make it to my doctor appointment the next morning. This time the snow was heavier because of the melt. A couple times, I had to pause to catch my breath. In the back of my mind, I had a nagging worry that something more serious was going on.

Monday morning I worked a couple hours, and then threw on a coat and drove to the cardiologist's office.

My cardiologist and I talked for a while and he wasn't sure what was going on with me. He was a little uncomfortable with a couple things, but not enough to be alarmed. Still he decided to do a full nuclear stress test. The first stage is to run a radioactive dye into your blood stream and then perform a scan. The second step is to exercise on a treadmill and then go back to the scanner.

On the treadmill, I began to get worried. At around 135 beats per minute, the heartburn started to come back and they went ahead and shut down the device.

Before I was done with the follow up scan, my doctor leaned over me and told me that he had already admitted me to the hospital. At that point, he wasn't sure how bad it was, but it was bad enough that they wanted me in the hospital leading up to a heart catheterization. He wasn't going to let me go home and didn't even want me to me to drive to the hospital, less than a mile away.

From there, things got very serious quickly. I got to call my wife and ask her to come get me. She wasn't thrilled with me for sending her a text at first. (Sorry, honey. Wasn't exactly a call I wanted to make.)I spent the night in the hospital and late the next afternoon, I went in for the heart catheterization. For this procedure, you are sedated, but not completely knocked out. In my case, they inserted a wire through my wrist and up into my heart. They were able to inject dye and see exactly where the problem areas were.

While I'd only had a little more than 24 hours to process all of this, I knew several people who had been through the same thing. I figured I had bought myself a couple stents. Immediately following the procedure, my doctor told me I had blockages and they were scheduling me for open-heart surgery.

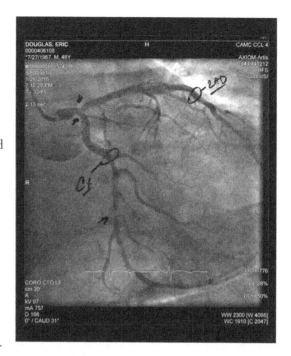

My mind began to reel. I was 48 years old. I had no family history of heart disease. Other than the occasional cigar, I've never smoked. All together I had five blockages ranging from 80 to 100 percent. There was also evidence that I had already had a heart attack.

Terms

So we're all on the same page, I want to define a couple terms I've used or that will come up later in this book. I don't intend this to be a medical textbook so if you have specific questions about your own situation or diagnosis, consult your doctor or one of the many online resources.

A heart attack is a situation where the blood supply to the heart muscle itself is cut off. Sometimes people imagine a heart attack is a restriction of the blood supply going through the heart, but that's not accurate. It is true, though, that a heart attack and the corresponding heart muscle damage can reduce blood flow to the rest of the body.

There are multiple blood vessels bringing oxygenated blood to the heart muscle. When they become blocked or restricted, sections of the heart muscle can be damaged or even die. When this happens, the heart stops working. Often, you will hear people refer to this as a "massive heart attack." More technically this is known as Sudden Cardiac Arrest. Damage to the heart muscle has become too great and the heart just quits. Heart muscle damage can also interfere with the electrical signals that tell the heart when and how fast to beat. When this happens, it may require a pacemaker or an implanted defibrillator to counteract the problem.

The amount of blood that flows out of the heart with each beat is referred to as Ejection Fraction. An ejection fraction of 55 to 75 percent is considered to be normal. That means 55 percent of the blood in the Left Ventricle is pushed out into the body with each beat. Damage to the heart muscle from a heart attack can reduce your ejection fraction making it hard for your body to get the oxygen and nutrients it needs.

A coronary artery bypass graft (CABG) is when a doctor takes a portion of a blood vessel from elsewhere in the body and uses it to jump over the blockage on the heart muscle. It is connected to the upstream side of the coronary artery and then connected past the blockage.

Hindsight

Looking back, I can see several places where I was having symptoms of heart trouble, but chose to ignore them.

More than once, mowing the grass, I had to squat down and "catch my breath."

Later in the fall, after we had some trees trimmed, I was moving logs and brush and had to sit down for a while even though I really hadn't been working that hard. At the time, I wrote it off as having smoked a cigar beforehand. That probably didn't help, but it wasn't the problem.

A couple times I jumped on the treadmill and only made it about 10 minutes before I had to stop because of the "heartburn."

Then, of course, is the heartburn attack following the boat parade before Christmas. Obviously, now I realize that was a heart attack. I remember squatting down to the floor, but still in my mind it was my stomach. I wouldn't accept that it was my heart. More importantly, in my mind at the time, my wife and daughters were there watching me, and I didn't want to upset them. What was I going to do? Go to the hospital right before Christmas? Of course, it has since been pointed out to me that I really would have ruined the holidays if I had died in the middle of them.

Every one of those instances is a case of denial. I knew the signs and symptoms of cardiac arrest, but I chose to ignore them. It couldn't be me. I was too young, too fit, too...

Except I wasn't.

As a quick refresher (according to the American Heart Association website):

- **Chest discomfort.** Most heart attacks involve discomfort in the center of the chest that lasts more than a few minutes, or that goes away and comes back. It can feel like uncomfortable pressure, squeezing, fullness or pain.

- **Discomfort in other areas of the upper body.** Symptoms can include pain or discomfort in one or both arms, the back, neck, jaw or stomach.

- **Shortness of breath** with or without chest discomfort.

- **Other signs** may include breaking out in a cold sweat, nausea or lightheadedness.

Women are somewhat more likely than men to experience some of the other common symptoms, particularly **shortness of breath, nausea/vomiting, and back or jaw pain**.

Again, in hindsight, I was overweight. I was sedentary. I ate too much fast food. I'm a writer and work from home. My job is to be at my computer even though I knew in my mind that my work would improve if I would get up and move. I had a treadmill in the next room, I felt guilty if I wasn't at my desk working.

Obviously, I have no idea what caused my arteries to block. It probably wasn't in the last year or two. Most likely, it built up over a long time. Still, I wasn't taking good care of myself and that sped the problem along.

Looking back, I am lucky I didn't drop over dead in my driveway while shoveling snow in the days leading up to my stress test. If I had had a heart attack, the EMS response would have been forever because the roads were blocked.

I denied a lot of symptoms in the months leading up to my heart attack and then the stress test and hospitalization. Ultimately, I got lucky. I know the stats on the survival for out-of-hospital cardiac arrest and they aren't good. I'm an advocate for CPR, but your chances of being resuscitated by bystander CPR are low. Like 5 to 10 percent low. [3]

If I had gone into cardiac arrest while mowing the lawn, shoveling snow or just walking through town, there is a good chance I wouldn't be here. Not with five blockages that ranged from 80 to 100 percent. My heart just wasn't working well enough.

Responses to the Survey

The following is a minimally-edited selection of diagnoses and reactions to the initial event. Many of these survivors describe situations where they didn't realize they were having a heart attack until the emergency room physician told them. Some are dramatic. Others are almost incidental.

Probably the most important lesson I took from reading these stories of diagnosis is there is no "typical" diagnosis or response to it. There is no typical patient, either. We are all individuals and unique. While warning signs are just that, one of the respondents was out training for a triathlon when it happened. Beyond that, one person said there were no symptoms, but he/she went to the emergency department four times before the heart issue was diagnosed. That means something was going on; there were symptoms, just not the typical ones. It's troubling that it took four trips to the emergency department, but at least he/she realized a problem existed and didn't deny it or try to ignore it.

Describe your diagnosis. When did it happen? What did your doctor tell you?

- Main left artery 99% blocked, plus an additional artery 75% blocked. No symptoms other than a mild pressure around chest area. I had a double bypass on New Year's Eve 2008.

- You know I never got an actual diagnosis that was named. It happened over the course of several days, but I guess the main event happened on a treadmill test the night I went to the ER. I had an 80% blockage in my left anterior descending (LAD) artery.

- During the first polar vortex--only sign was slight chest pain when I walked my dog. I thought it was from the cold weather because the pain wouldn't last long and I didn't feel pain while indoors.

- At age 45, I had a widow-maker heart attack. I had a 5x Coronary Artery Bypass Graft (CABG). Four arteries were 100% clogged and one was 85%. My cardiologist told me I was extremely lucky to be alive.

- Had a migraine for weeks. Did stress tests, angiogram and landed on the operating table for quadruple bypass at age 50.

- I had experienced extreme jaw pain one night coming home from work. By the time I arrived home, the pain was down my left arm and I was disoriented. I knew something was very wrong. I was taken to the ER and they found nothing wrong but referred me to a cardiologist the next day. I spent three days with him running tests, with no conclusions. Every time I walked more than about 20 feet the crushing jaw pain returned. On the fourth day, I had an angiogram. Unbeknownst to the cardiologist, I had a tear inside my right main artery. The catheter caught the tear and ripped the artery completely open, along with an adjoining one. I suffered a massive heart attack in the cath lab and died for several minutes. I remember the heart attack - it was terrifying. I felt paralyzed, unable to speak, intense heat, unable to breathe... I knew I was dying. People were shouting, alarms going off. I remember. And then I was gone. (I have been dealing with PTSD for three years now. It is slowly improving.) After many chest compressions, nitro injections into my heart, and two paddle shocks, I came back. The doctor told my 17-year-old daughter what had happened and told her the only way to fix it was to do an emergent double bypass with CABG. They also told her I had less than a 10% chance of surviving. But I made it. I woke up the next day and was told what happened.

- I was 41, quite healthy. I had a heart attack - chest pain and numb arms. I had no clue I was having heart attack. I was admitted to hospital and after three days, I was scheduled for angiogram. While doing the test, my arteries were ruptured and I was rushed to the op room and there, I had triple bypass. I was opened for 4 days and was losing a lot of blood. I was alive with the machine.

- I had a little poking feeling in the middle of my chest. Not really painful but uncomfortable. This started on a Wednesday, on

Thursday I went to my PCP. He ran an EKG and did an exam. Everything looked great. So he sent me for blood work and to a Cardiologist on Friday morning. I did my lab work first thing in the morning, then went to the cardiologist that afternoon. The cardiologist did an EKG, a sonogram, and after what seemed like a few minutes, told me "you are just fat, and need to exercise, go home and come back in two weeks!" At 7pm, I got a call from my PCP office, the nurse told me the protein level in my heart was extremely elevated and I needed to call 911 and go to the hospital via ambulance.

- It was a surprise...ended up in emergency where the Emergency Doctor tried to get the heart attack under control. Didn't work so I was transported to a larger hospital where they did an angiogram. From 911 call to bypass surgery was 8 hours.

- Woke up in a hospital bed in Texas and was told I had a stroke.

- No heart attack. No symptoms. Kept going back to ER (4 times) & each time they did blood, etc. tests & told me I was OK. 4th time I persuaded a stress test. Failed. Precipitated a dye test. Failed (2 @ 90% blocked, 3rd @ 40%). Quick triple bypass. Recovery went well (only recovering from surgery, not a heart attack).

- Coronary Artery Disease, 100 percent blockage in the LAD. Doctor told me nothing but I needed a stent. I was terrified. Had the heart attack in 2012.

- Was out training for triathlon, fainted, taken to hospital, no defect found. Follow up investigations revealed 3 blocked arteries. It was obvious from the angiogram. Further tests showed no heart damage.

- I saw four different cardiologists. The first said I had a pulmonary problem, the second said I had an Autonomic Nervous System disorder. The third confirmed the 2nd. I told the fourth the same issue after 5 years of problems and he got it right and just in time. Within two months of seeing the fourth doctor I narrowly avoided a heart attack and was having quintuple bypass surgery. As an avid cyclist I saw my heart rate under a workload become lower and lower over a 5+ year period. The fourth cardiologist, also a cyclist, did the right tests and interpreted them correctly. I was sent for angioplasty in April 2011 but upon inspection was scheduled the following day for the bypass. I still cycle though I have never returned to the level I enjoyed and that is including the aging process.

- Mini-stroke at 47. Heart attack at 49. I drove myself to the doctor after symptoms of mini-stroke continued over the weekend. Was told I had to be admitted to the hospital on Monday by my doctor. Spent 4 days being observed and tested. Recovered in two weeks and had physical therapy on my right hand for a month. At 49, I had discomfort in my chest all day which worsened by the next morning. Drove myself to the hospital where I spent 16 hours being tested. Finally admitted and in a cath lab the next morning. Found a 99 percent blockage of my circumflex but damage was already done. I have severe mitral valve regurgitation which will eventually have to be fixed or replaced.

- I was 48. Drove myself to ER having a heart attack. Next morning, they did heart cath then came to waiting area and told my family I was probably not going to live. They had to take me into surgery with cath still in my heart. I had 3 critical blockages. They were 100%. Rear chamber of my heart had no blood in it and was shriveled up. Doctor has no explanation as to why I was still alive. That was 2 years ago, and I'm still on the path to my old self.

- Diagnosis is coronary artery disease. Had "woman's/silent heart attack". I was sure it wasn't a heart attack, but made an appointment with a cardiologist just in case. One stress test later, I was in the cath lab with 3 stents in my LAD. About a year passed, then those "feelings" started to be noticeable. Nuclear stress test... and I'm back in the cath lab. Can't be cathed, so on to CABG x4 (4-1-2016). 6 months later, feeling odd again. Another nuclear stress test, and another trip to the cath lab (11-28-2016) for 2 stents in Right Coronary Artery. LAD looks good. 2 other bypasses are 40-50% blocked. Angles make them hard to stent.

- Coronary heart disease. I was diagnosed in August 2016 when I went to the ER after 8 hours (overnight) of a combination of chest pressure, diarrhea, vomiting, severe sweating, neck & back pain. I didn't think it was a heart attack, so I didn't rush to the hospital & instead waited until the morning (I was VERY lucky!). I was told that I had 100% blockage of my left main (or widow-maker) after they tried to do an angioplasty. I was told I'd need open-heart surgery for a bypass. My heart attack was caused by a clot, which may have been caused by an auto immune disease. I'm waiting for an appointment with a rheumatologist to confirm that.

- When I woke in the morning at about 0630, I had a severe crushing pain in my chest, my Doctor sent me straight to Emergency where they treated me where subsequently was admitted into the Cardiac Care Unit and was told that I had Myocardial Infarction.

- Essentially heart failure due to genetics. Triple bypass. September 8 @ about 9 a.m. Doc said due to my health status (great other than my heart) I should recover with minimal impact.

- Massive heart attack. No symptoms, just vomiting. 3 x 100% blocks caused by blood clots. Took me 3 days to realize that the vomiting wasn't just caused by a virus. Massive heart damage.

- "I gave up smoking and was on Chantix. Started getting chest pain that would last for a minute or so then I would feel the amazing euphoria when the pain passed. Went back to the doctor a few times and they just kept giving me more medication for indigestion as that was a side effect from the Chantix. This went on for 6 weeks. I woke up one morning about 2 am with the Pain and it didn't go away.... long story short I had a 100% blockage of the right coronary artery. Stent fitted.

- Was sick and nauseous after hiking sand dunes. Went to urgent care thinking it was an allergic reaction. Sent me to ER and I had two 100% blockages in the LAD. Ejection Fraction (EF) has not improved from 20-25 in one year. Have an implantable cardioverter defibrillator (ICD) now.

- Pressure dead center of chest. Intense profuse sweating. Triage thought anxiety. EKG said heart attack. Cardiologist said 80% mortality rate. I was lucky I went in when I did. 10/28/2016.

- I was diagnosed with a Spontaneous Coronary Artery Dissection (SCAD) heart attack. I was over 90% blocked with blood in my LAD which meant I needed a double bypass!! My artery had dissected.

- Felt odd and had a headache. He was a pilot and was getting ready to fly so he went to his Doctor. They sent him to the ER and they did a cath and found a blockage. While trying to dissolve and remove it, the blockage shattered and it hit the right side of his brain. They stroked him out on the table. The recovery continues but the damage is permanent.

- I had a heart attack New Year's Day 2016....this led to a discovery of major blockages and eventual quintuple bypass surgery four days later.

- I had a family history on both sides of cardiac arrest. I had minor indications via EKG of problems 12 years ago. Drugs, diet and exercise slowed it a bit, but after two years I needed bypasses.

- Ischemic stroke. No warning or risk factor. It happened at night while having a migraine. Doctors can only point at the migraines for being the cause.

Chapter 4: Surgery

My experience with surgery

Once my cardiologist told me that I had blockages and was scheduling me for surgery, I felt a bit like I was being carried along in a river. I didn't feel out of control, but it did feel like there wasn't a lot I could do about it. The diagnosis put procedures into motion and I was just along for the ride.

Oddly, though, I never felt uncomfortable or scared. In some ways, it was reassuring that they did the surgery often enough that there was an entire system in place.

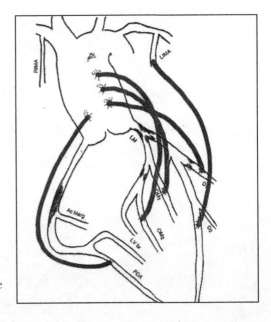

I had to wait two full days before my surgery. They said they like to have patients in the hospital for a couple days, if it's not an emergency, to get some medications in your system and that sort of thing. Those days were tedious for me. I had nothing to do except wait. I did have my laptop with me and so I did some work while sitting in my hospital room. Several friends came by to see me and I appreciated that distraction as well.

In theory, I understood what was going to happen. I knew they were going to take veins from my leg to bypass the arteries providing blood to my heart. I knew they were going to have to crack my chest open and that was going to take a while to heal. The night before the surgery, my wife strongly suggested I watch the informational video on the hospital channel about the surgery. It was only then that it occurred to me that they were going to have to stop my heart to make all of this happen. I don't know why that thought never crossed my mind. It makes perfect sense, but I never stopped to consider it. My friend Bob Wohlers, who has been through open-heart surgery twice, refers to this as "having your heart exposed to air." Again, it makes perfect sense until you suddenly realize it is your heart they are stopping and exposing to air.

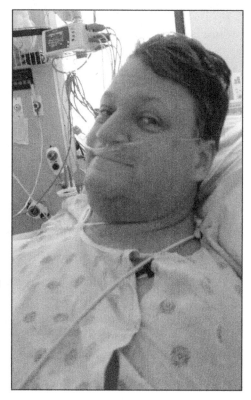

The morning of surgery was easy for me. I mean, I just had to lay there. I didn't have to set an alarm or anything. They came and got me. They weighed me and then took me away. A friend from high school happened to work in surgery and he coordinated my surgical team. He said it was the team he would want doing his surgery. After that, the anesthesiologist did his job and I slept.

By all accounts, my surgery went as expected. No complications. I spent about a day in Coronary Intensive Care. That period is pretty much a blur. I remember the nurse caring for me saying something about me trying to bite him, but I think it was related to my endotracheal tube. Other than that, I blame it on the anesthesia.

Coming home

I was so ready to go home when the doctors finally gave me permission. Not that I stayed in an unusual amount of time or anything. I had surgery on Friday and was released on Wednesday. And I have no complaints about the care I received. Everyone did their best to take care of me. It was simply the idea that being in the hospital wasn't home. I wanted to be comfortable. And most importantly, I wanted to begin my recovery process. I knew that wouldn't really start until I was on my own.

Just before I was discharged, a woman from the cardiac rehab program stopped by. I think I surprised her a little bit when I immediately said I was ready to sign up for rehab. She didn't have to convince me. Too many friends had told me, or sent me notes, that it was the best thing I could do. What did surprise me was that she gave me some home rehab work to do. The official cardiac rehab wouldn't start for about a month, but they wanted me up and walking the very next day.

I have a home treadmill so there was no problem with being able to walk for exercise. The first couple days, they wanted me to walk for six minutes, three or four times a day. The first day, I walked for six minutes, took a nap and then walked another six minutes. It was all I could do. I was totally exhausted. Another time, just a few days later, following my second or third walk, I decided to go straight to the shower that happens to be on the same floor as the treadmill. I almost passed out in the shower.

Lesson learned: regardless of how strong you used to be, it's going to take a few days to get everything working right again. Your heart might be working better now, with improved blood flow, but it's not used to it and neither is anything else.

I referred to those days as trudging. I would sit in my easy chair and nap or work or watch television and then go downstairs to trudge on the treadmill. I was literally going 1.5 miles an hour in those early days.

I wish I could say my recovery was linear. In the big picture, it probably was. I have steadily increased my stamina and strength since January 29, 2016. My resting heart rate and blood pressure are lower. I am up to a consistent jogging pace at more than five miles per hour, much better than my mile and a half an hour pace. Close up, though, there were good days and bad days. Some days I felt stronger and would push it a bit. The next day, I would still be paying for it and have to slow it down, take it easy or I would take a longer nap. I'm sure that is totally normal. I tried to keep telling myself that, but there were days it was frustrating.

At my hospital, and I've been told that others do the same thing, they gave me a heart-shaped pillow (you see it on the book cover). This served a couple different purposes. It has a silk-screen image of a real heart with the major blood vessels on it. My doctor used a Sharpie to draw in the bypasses. It was great for me to explain to others exactly what had happened.

More importantly, the pillow provides you something to hold on to. Having your sternum sawed in half causes a lot of pain. Every time you move, it hurts. Coughing really hurts. Sneezing is awful. Clutching that pillow to your chest when you are getting up, about to cough, or if you have the time to grab it, before you sneeze makes it less excruciating.

A few hours a day, I would go downstairs to my desk and sit at my computer for a while. I could move my laptop upstairs to my recliner, but it felt good to sit up and feel like I was getting back to normal. One day, after

I had been home a couple weeks, I sneezed. My wife Beverly was still upstairs and she heard the sneeze and then she heard me groan. She realized it was my first sneeze and my pillow was still upstairs. I did a better job of keeping it with me after that.

Chapter 5: Accepting Help

Letting others help

Aside from the nearly dying while shoveling snow thing, it was probably to my advantage that most of this happened in the winter. I am an active person. I like to be busy. If I had been confined to the house, or my easy chair, in the summer, it probably would have driven me crazy.

As it was, February was cold and rainy/snowy and March wasn't much better. I stayed inside, exercised and napped without feeling guilty.

Aside from being unable to get out much, one of the biggest stumbling blocks for me was letting other people do things for me. At my home, I do most of the cooking. That was one of the first places where I had to let someone else help me. My wife Beverly stepped up and cooked, but she was faced with two challenges. She really hadn't cooked much since we had gotten married four years before, so she was out of practice and really didn't even know where a lot of the utensils were. The second challenge for her was we wanted to go ahead and start cooking in a heart-healthy fashion, so she was trying to cook and figure out new things to cook. She did a great job.

In the winter, I like to keep a fire in the fireplace. We don't need it to heat the house, but it is a nice supplemental heat. The hearth is in the family room where my desk is and it makes it nice to go work with a fire at your back. But, of course, I wasn't permitted to move firewood around. I had the post-surgery/10-pound weight limit on things I could lift or move and that did not include bringing in an armload of firewood. I had to ask two friends, JD and Mike from across the street, to come and move firewood for me. Both did it graciously and without complaint.

I was 48 when I had my surgery. That meant I had been driving for more than two-thirds of my life. Suddenly being told I couldn't drive was a bit of an indignity. I read one of the survey respondents say that he/she drove exactly two weeks after surgery. I doubt I would have been up to that. My doctor had me wait a full month after my surgery and while it was frustrating, it was probably best. I remember being tired after taking my first short drive post-surgery. My sternum was still healing and was especially sensitive. Raising my arms to the steering wheel and twisting to look over my shoulder hurt. Until my doctor cleared me to drive, I wasn't getting behind the wheel. Beverly drove me wherever I needed to go.

As we got into spring, the grass started growing up and my yard was getting shaggy. I was feeling better, although I was likely not up to mowing my grass yet. It didn't matter though, because the doctor hadn't released me to do any heavy lifting and Beverly wasn't hearing any of it when I suggested I could lift more, or push the mower. My next-door neighbor, Paul, who is about 20 years older than I am, mowed my grass for me. A couple times. I really appreciated him doing that, but it was hard to swallow.

It's a hard balance to strike. Your family wants to help you out and your friends are more than happy to help you, too. But you want to do things for yourself and don't want to be babied. I made the best of it, but it was a challenge. Beverly was happy for me to take over the cooking duties as soon as I felt up to it.

In rehab, I remember a man talking about how frustrated he got that his family wouldn't let him do anything at all. It was causing him a fair amount of stress. They were trying so hard to help him, but for him it was having the opposite effect.

Responses to the Survey

The following is a minimally-edited selection of help survivors received from others. The responses range from family, to friends to support groups and Facebook groups. This is an important piece for not only survivors, but family members to understand. The most common responses were that family provided reassurance and encouragement. Most survivors don't need much more than that. They need someone to be there and tell them they can do it. It also helps to get a reminder from time to time that you are changing your lifestyle and putting in the hard work for more than just yourself.

The second most important take-away from this is it helps if you aren't making changes in a vacuum. Having your family eat the same foods you do, for your health and theirs, for example makes it seem less like you are going on a diet and more like a change for life. When your family is there to work with you, walk with you and help you, it makes all the difference in the world.

That said, there are people out there who live alone, or as one survivor said, "I am a loner." It is still important to make those changes and keep living. It just takes more determination to make the changes. Online support groups, or support groups offered through the hospital and cardiac rehab are valuable in the recovery process. Again, there is no single way to get through this. If you don't have a support system at home, find one elsewhere. Just never give up.

Can you offer an example of the help you received from others?

- Prayer and reassurance during a time I felt alone and depressed.

- Encouragement and support when I am down.

- Help with taking care of my dog.

- My wife now only cooks Whole Foods Plant-Based Diet meals and I do exhaustive reading and research on this topic.

- I'm a loner, so I did it 99% myself. Family added to the stress factor.

- My husband was absolutely my rock for not only the physical assistance but also the mental. The therapist at cardiac rehab were there for me as well for both physical and mental struggles.

- I really think the help I received was being scared to death from having a heart attack. That was the reality and the catalyst for change. There was no thinking twice about it; I was scared. I did not want this to happen again. So, change happened. It was like a switch went off.

- I found help from Facebook groups of similar diagnosis.

- Kept plugging and was complimented by the teachers.

- Wife driving me to good places to walk and good diet food.

- Support groups. My kids and friends were worthless on this.

- A friend and my wife who are personal trainers. Friends and my wife for taking up running and biking with me.

- I am in a demanding job and upper management told me to do whatever I need to get back to a full recovery.

- They helped me to get a routine and hopeful of a future.

- Confidence, support, programs for training, controlled environment for rehab taught me to have some faith in my body.

- Wife's constant care & support plus my own obsessive interest in fixing my lousy cardiac genealogy.

- Honestly never got much help.

- It was all about encouragement, my wife bought me a $3000 mountain bike for motivation for example.

- I stayed with my sister for the first month after surgery and my other sister (RN) and my daughter (RN) came to help. The Rehab nurse kept me from going overboard but knew I could be challenged much more than a patient who had a heart attack and allowed me to do more than normal.

- I have received no help other than financial so I am not homeless due to health/bills. They expect me to just get over it and return to normal.

- Phone calls and help when needed.

- Brother helped with shopping and talking.

- Getting the best support coming from your family because that is the second-best support you can get. Most importantly, make sure you have a close relationship with God. Prayers work.

- Healthy Heart program at hospital was wonderful for encouraging exercise and providing information to make sense out of it. Counselor helped me emotionally. Sister and my kids were concerned and helped me with household tasks and transportation during rehab. My work helped by having limited duty and easing my transition back to work.

- Gift of an excellent plant-based diet book. Facebook group called The Zipper Club.

- The only person I had at home was my daughter - she did everything from food shopping to cooking, to helping me shower and slowly get over my fear of falling, to making sure I had my meds on time.

- Encouragement and walking with me. Helping me keep track of my fluid/salt intake and eating healthier with me.

- My wife and I stopped eating red meat and began eating lots of vegies and fruit.

- They continue to recognize the weight I've lost and changes of bad habits.

- Partner fully supports healthy lifestyle changes. She does all the food preparation and has done a lot of research about nutrition. Entire family often goes for fast walks together.

- Constant support and advice on what to eat, and what not to, because my daughter wants me alive.

- Husband very willing to make dietary changes. Help and patience at home.

- My husband has been there 100% and l couldn't have done it without him. Friends are sympathetic but don't understand. My parents helped me tremendously when I first came home. From helping to feed my dog, to my mom even helping me take a bath because I wasn't able to on my own at that time. As time passed friends & family offered lots of support. I got ALOT of cards from friends, which I've kept as encouragement on the days when I felt tired or achy.

- I have a very good family and friend support group. My wife has been amazingly strong and resilient, despite her health issues. I have a friend who comes weekly to be a partner in exercise.

- Social workers such as community care nurse. Ongoing government subsidized home cleaning because I can't do that now. I had to fight a very difficult battle to get DSP which took 2.5 years.

- I admin several Facebook support pages and a heart healthy cooking page. I find talking to others around the world with the same problems helps a lot.

- They were so scared that they took such good care of me. No fighting amongst the teens, no cooking dinner for them, they did all the laundry, they paid someone to clean the house! My friends took me to movies so I could get out of the house. They cooked my family dinner every night for 3 weeks after I got home from the hospital. The list goes on and on! My employees went above and beyond too.

- My whole family has changed their eating habits.

- My ex and my sister don't smoke when I'm around. My 7-year-old told me she's proud of me for quitting smoking. That strengthened my resolve to stay healthy.

- Making meals for me. Taking me to Doctor appointments. Helping me with household chores.

- My boyfriend has been helping me with my children. My sister helps with errands. My best friend either calls or texts every day to check in on me. My neighbors check in too. They know I can't shovel snow or lift heavy things anymore.

- Encouragement and allowing me to talk about how I felt.

- The cardiac rehab staff gave me the positive feedback I needed to gain confidence and push myself when I was afraid to. New friends that I made in the rehab program also set a good example and made the program enjoyable.

- Regularly walking as a family.

- Although our kids are out of state they call on a regular basis. My wife lays out my medication and see that I take them daily. She is a very strong person and wants me around for another 53 years.

- A place to recover and reside. He lost everything when he couldn't work: home, plane, vehicle, RV, two businesses. Without Katrina who knows what would have happened.

- Support: many encouragements on Facebook while in recovery. Rehab folks very attentive and suggestive on advice, home health care nurse very positive.

- People came to the house and hospital to help my husband care for me during the worst of it.

Chapter 6: Setbacks

Relapse

About a month after I came home from the hospital, I wasn't feeling right. I felt like there were times I couldn't breathe and there was a pain in my chest. My heart rate was okay, but something felt wrong.

Considering how many times I had denied trouble leading up to being hospitalized in the first place, I decided not to risk it. I told my wife we needed to go to the emergency room.

Honestly, when I told them I had recently had open-heart surgery, I expected to be whisked off to the back room somewhere. In a sense I was. They quickly checked me out and determined I wasn't an emergency case. After that, things slowed down quite a bit.

I won't belabor the point of this return visit to the hospital too much. I ended up spending the night and they ran an entire battery of tests on me, including a chemical stress test. Ultimately, they determined that I had the appearances of early stage pneumonia. This was probably brought on by post-anesthesia and not breathing all that deeply because of the pain in my chest.

My guess is there was an ample amount of post-surgical paranoia mixed in there, too. My father-in-law had bypass surgery several years ago, before I knew him, and one or more of his bypasses collapsed. They ended up having to give him stents, too. I worried that was happening to me.

The good news about this was the chemical stress test, the ultrasound and every other test they ran showed that my heart was in great shape and had recovered to the high end of normal ejection fraction.

The important lesson to learn from this for me was that I had to adjust to a new normal with my body. I was used to my body feeling and reacting one way, but I had to learn what the new way was going to be. There was something wrong for me, but it wasn't my heart. I also had to know that it wasn't acceptable for me to deny or put things off any more.

Responses to the Survey

The following is a minimally-edited selection of comments from survivors about setbacks they faced during their recovery. Many people identified psychological setbacks as well as physical ones. The most important lesson from this survey question is everyone has set backs. They are inevitable. Just don't let those setbacks derail your recovery. The last comment sums it up. "I stayed focused on my goal."

Understanding that life has thrown you a curve ball is important. There will be a new normal. You just have to keep fighting and working to improve. If you stumble, have a bad food day, or don't work out for three or four days, you just accept it and move on. Long-term goals make this easier. Another important lesson is to remember that it is never too late to start. A couple respondents said they had trouble losing weight and nearly gave up, or were "recovery failures" until their doctor told them to investigate gastric bypass surgery. Even nine years later, you can make changes to improve your health.

Setbacks are inevitable when making lifestyle changes. It is a marathon, not a sprint. Everyone gets frustrated or tired and wants to

give up at some point. Did you hit any roadblocks during your recovery? What were those roadblocks and what did you do to overcome them?

- Other health problems gave me many setbacks. Add in the depression, anxiety and lack of sleep and well I still haven't gotten there, but I will.

- I could not lose weight no matter what I did. After much struggling my cardiologist insisted I see a surgeon for gastric bypass because I should have been losing weight and wasn't.

- Lack of support from my spouse.

- Anxiety, learning how to read my body's messages (learning how to trust). Talk to wife and brother about feelings and symptoms, visit emergency room when felt necessary.

- Mostly mental it was hard to accept the fact that it was hard work and I try not to but I still fall down. I plan on getting into a pool at my local gym Monday.

- I lost 70 pounds and then gained 50 back. Lost my motivation.

- Yes, one of my bypasses has a kink so had to work around getting angina when exercising.

- My roadblocks are mental. High anxiety and a diagnosis of Generalized Anxiety Disorder from Post-Traumatic Stress Disorder. I am taking a low dose of SSRI Escitalopram and starting therapy soon.

- I had none. My amazing wife Freda knows a lot about nutrition, is an amazing cook and after the surgery I listened to her more attentively and acted on her advice.

- Depression and anxiety made me want to give up, I turn to heart attack survivor websites so I get some inspiration.

- None really. I was slowed down initially because I was worried the artery connections would fail with exertion. I knew it would be a slow recovery, I did a lot of walking, 6-10 miles per day, before converting that to jogging and then running. Also, got back on the bike almost immediately. I never really had any physical setbacks. I think I was lucky as I was fit (not healthy) going into surgery and bounced back quickly and relatively painlessly.

- Mental illness (PTSD among others) has made this more difficult than I think it should be.

- Yes. It does not always seem easy to eat healthy and exercise. Just keep going one day at a time. I have a 12-year-old. I want to be here for him.

- I went through anxiety and depression. I took meds, attended counseling with our psychologist, got regular exercise, and learned a new hobby.

- Fatigue was and remains a roadblock to me. As time passes, my energy level has gradually increased, but has never reached the before surgery level. I have realized that this is just what I have to live with, my new normal. With acceptance of this new normal, I have changed how I do things and ceased to do others.

- Truthfully, I'm at a roadblock now. I am separated 14 months from a 40-year long marriage and I'm struggling daily.

- Rehabilitation was not easy, it took time to recover. I was always scared to do things. I begin to make activities that help me to heal the mind.

- Mostly had trouble getting my strength back and had a lot of trouble with fluid retention and trouble breathing. Kept asking my doctor questions and leaned on my husband to offer support.

- Oh, yes, I did. I have a serious large herniation in my lower back. I had to stop walking due to the severe pain in my legs and back.

- Not really. I have a support group, just guys my age that I've met at the gym. Attending makes me feel good about myself.

- Quitting tobacco. I have used substitutes and have stayed strong.

- During my separation from my husband and financial issues that occurred, the stress was bad. I did slip a few times and smoke. I had to find another outlet to handle stress.

- A lot of pain especially at the site of the chest tubes (after they were removed).

- The pain of the surgical aftermath. Knowing when I had chest pain if it was surgery or heart pain. Also, people think you will be normal again.

- Fear of getting sick again and lots of uncontrollable emotions. I had to work through it with lots of prayer and positive thoughts.

- Main roadblock, mentally and physically, was having angina pains and ending up being cathed again less than eight months after CABG x4! I am still dealing with this since I had stents placed 5 days ago. Starting with baby steps. Test the waters so to speak. Started with grocery trip with hubby this evening. Tomorrow we will go on my first long walk.

- I was laid up for about two months so my biggest obstacle was having to learn to walk again and living in a two-story town home sleeping in my own bed was very important.

- There were several things I couldn't do right away, even as simple as making my bed or opening a jar. But I knew that one day I'd be able to and that I would just need help for the moment to get to where I need to be. I learned to be very patient with myself.

- Initially there was mild depression. I attribute this to medical rather than psychological components. I've never been a "Why me" person. I felt it was a question of time to regain being positive and proactive. I was right and continue to push my rehab, within the proper boundaries.

- I lost 50 pounds, but my diet and exercise are a daily struggle. Also, my meds are hard on my body - always tired and sore from the statins. I just suck it up and try and deal with it.

- My rehab start date was delayed two months because another heart problem popped up. I was hospitalized for arterial fibrillation and put on medication for that. It was scarier than the bypass surgery, because my heart stopped during one of the episodes. I really wanted to get started with the rehab program to have supervised exercise as I tried to get fit again.

- At times, I became depressed because we were no longer going to Florida in the winter. I had a very strong-willed wife who kept me motivated.

- Frustration over limitations. Reminding myself of progress and that while I was slower than desired I was still alive.

- Learning to live with limits. Continue therapy and meds.

- I just found out it is a slower process than I had hoped; months of recovery instead of weeks. Dizzy spells due to summer heat.

- Aphasia is the worst roadblock, but it is slowly getting better. My inability to use my right arm after my stroke is hard, but with adaptive equipment I'm able to drive again.

- I just never lost focus. I hit walls or things didn't happen as quickly as I wanted, but I never quit. I stayed focused on my goal.

Chapter 7: Going Public

Charleston Gazette-Mail

Talking about heart disease helps others

By Eric Douglas

March 16, 2016

My friend Jean calls it living life out loud.

She means talking about what is going on in your life so others can benefit from your experiences. That doesn't mean airing your dirty laundry on Facebook to get attention. In my case, if you've been following along recently, you know it means talking about heart disease and my own experiences with open-heart surgery, recovery and cardiac rehab.

Probably the funniest response to one of these columns was from my heart surgeon. I went in for a follow-up a few days ago. After he checked me out and gave me his seal of approval, he asked how my first column about heart disease (titled: "Don't Make the Same Mistake I Did") appeared in the paper the same day he released me from the hospital. I told him I had been bored in my hospital bed. I had time to write.

I've really enjoyed hearing from others who have had similar experiences. Many of the people who've sent me notes or emails have had great advice or encouragement to offer. The coolest part of talking about it though is realizing I've made a difference in someone else's life. While not unheard of, needing five bypasses at 48 years of age is somewhat unusual. By writing about my situation, others who are close to me in age, or even younger with some family history or other risk factors, are realizing that they aren't immune to heart disease and need to get themselves checked out. Because of my experiences, they are calling their doctors and going in for a physical or a stress test.

"Cousin Bill" got a clean bill of health from his doctor, Gene was scheduling a stress test and Chris, a friend since high school, sent me an email to tell me that he was planning major changes to his own lifestyle and meeting with his doctor to get approval for his plan.

I also got a very nice letter from a new friend named Dick who had bypass surgery several years ago and received a stent just a few weeks ago. Now, Dick is preparing to leave on a long vacation in his RV. He closed his letter with this thought: "The road has not been smooth, but we make the most of what time the Good Lord gives us."

If by living my life out loud (when it comes to heart disease) I can help a few people live longer and "make the most of what time the Good Lord gives us," I've done my job.

Going public

You may have seen stories where a photographer facing brain cancer decided to document everything, for example. I've always thought to myself that if I were put into that situation, I would hope I would so the same. Talking about a situation like that, going public with it, serves to encourage others to act or get themselves checked or to make changes in their own life.

I'm a fair photographer, but there are a lot of people much better than me. After thinking about it, I wasn't sure I could do this justice with a camera. The other reason I decided to write about this whole process rather than try to photograph it was, from my perspective, open-heart surgery would be a relatively short procedure with a long recovery and rehabilitation. I didn't feel that lent itself to a visual project.

I also wanted something that I could begin publishing and talking about immediately. I knew my story was unusual, but at the same time typical. There are lots of men and women my age who aren't caring for themselves as they should, who don't have obvious risk factors, but still could use some encouragement to talk to their doctors and to make some changes in their lives.

For the last several years, I have written a weekly column for my local newspaper. It runs in the hometown news/Metro section and isn't one of the official editorial page columns. Because of that, they let me talk about pretty much anything I want. I decided that would be an ideal location to start talking about my situation. (You've read several, although not all, of the columns I wrote as I recovered.)

I also write a regular monthly column for Scuba Diving Magazine. From my hospital bed, I sent the editors an email asking if they would be interested in a series of articles for their website about recovering from open-heart surgery. I knew a fair number of divers faced the same situation and I thought my recovery would give them inspiration. They accepted and I began writing a monthly series. That series has a scuba diving focus, but if you are interested in reading it, you can find the links on the Diving and Heart Disease page on my website booksbyeric.com or by going to .ScubaDiving.com. I received cards, letters, emails and phone calls from all of it.

A good friend of mine, Greg Holt, checked in with me immediately when he heard about my situation. Once the first ScubaDiving.com column went online, Greg invited me on his syndicated radio talk show to discuss my situation and recovery. ScubaRadio™ is broadcast on radio stations across the country and he has a significant online following, both live and as podcast downloads.

Greg had me on the show several times over the next several months to talk about how I was feeling and what I was learning, as well as how long it would take me to recover and return to diving.

Just as I was finishing up my recovery and getting cleared to dive, Greg called me to let me know he was following in my footsteps. He had just failed a stress test and was scheduled for bypass surgery, too. Greg said he felt much better prepared for what he was facing because he had talked to me about my situation so much. He knew what the surgery would be like, what he needed to do and how long it would take him to get back underwater.

Greg made the same decision I did and has been very outspoken about his condition and his recovery as well. He has had numerous people contact him to say that hearing his story encouraged them to visit their doctor and get checked out. Several have even said they found blockages and are getting the help they needed to improve their health.

If it hadn't been for Greg talking about his situation and encouraging others to visit their doctors, it is entirely possible some of those people might not be here today. They easily could have had a heart attack and not made it to the hospital.

In 2016, there were more than 350,000 out-of-hospital cardiac arrests, according to the American Heart Association website. Bystanders delivered CPR 46 percent of the time, but the survival rate (to discharge from the hospital) was only 12 percent. That number has increased slightly over the last few years, but only slightly. That means 308,000 didn't come home from the hospital after having a heart attack.

Not everyone can write for an international magazine or to talk about heart disease from their radio show, but simply telling your story might save the life of someone you love by encouraging them to talk to a doctor as well. I can't think of any better use of this experience than that. On the other hand, don't become a zealot. I've seen more than one person go through open-heart surgery and become "holier-than-thou" about their recovery. They view anyone who hasn't made all the same changes they have made as inferior or weak. They spout off constantly why everything they are doing is the best way and that everyone else is wrong. That attitude doesn't help anyone.

Responses to the Survey

The following is a minimally-edited selection of reactions to the diagnosis. The news that you have had a heart attack or that you are facing open-heart surgery can be difficult to take. Totally understandably, the overall reactions are fear and shock and then worrying about loved ones.

Describe your feelings when the doctor told you there was a problem.

- Shocked.
- Scared, freaked out. I went in for a stent and during the procedure

my cardiologist told me no stent and that I would need surgery the next day.

- Amazement.

- Disappointed.

- Fear!

- Thankful I was still alive.

- I knew it was a heart attack before doctor told me. Shock and disbelief. I had always been extremely healthy.

- Bottom fell out of my world.

- A positive feeling of a problem going to be fixed.

- It scared me. I was unable to speak.

- Disbelief. I thought it was my gallbladder.

- I was scared and thought "I am doomed."

- I was worried for my family.

- It was so sudden I didn't have time to react.

- Total disbelief, had to be a mistake.

- I woke up from surgery in ICU and was told everything by my doctor. I was in shock and pissed off at myself for letting my health get that bad.

- I immediately thought of my children, who are grown, but still needed me. I thought "I'm too young to die." I didn't have much time to think of anything else and it was over.

- Disbelief at first, then some anger. I inherited a bad heart from my father. Felt I was far too young at 59 to face these issues considering I had always been in very good health.

- When I was told I needed a triple bypass, I said, "Okay. When can you do it?" He said tomorrow. When I was wheeled back into my hospital room, I cried for about 5 minutes thinking it was my fault, but then that passed and I was very calm.

- I was shocked because I'm only 36 and although heart disease is in my family, it's a generation removed. I've always had good blood pressure and cholesterol. I never smoked, or did drugs, I drank only socially and I ate pretty healthy (I eat much healthier now). I did feel like I had a guardian angel with me and that sense of presence calmed me a lot. It's hard to explain, but I know that my cousin's late husband was with me. He suffered a heart attack & seizure just three months prior, but didn't make it. He was 33.

- Can't repeat that language!

- Shock, utter shock. I asked the urgent care doc if I would make it and he gave me a grim look. In the ER, I heard some tech saying "Did you see her ECG?" Then they sent a chaplain in!

- I thought they were nuts the first time. I felt like I slept on my arm wrong.

- I was petrified!! And broke down in tears!! But I was reassured that I would sail through the operation.

- I was scared to death. My boyfriend took me to the ER and all I could think of was when I could go home to be with my kids.

- I was surprised because I hadn't had any previous issues with shortness of breath and didn't have any chest pain. I expected that I would get stents put in and was upset when I was told bypass was necessary. I didn't see any alternatives at the time, and went ahead with the surgery.

- Depressed for about 3 minutes and then resolved to work it.

- For twelve years, I complained and was told it was not my heart, so it was shocking that it in fact was my heart. When I learned that

I needed bypass surgery I was dismayed for about an hour, then I figured I had no option so I got psyched up to get through it.

Chapter 8: Changes

Charleston Gazette-Mail

Being heart-healthy means simple changes

By Eric Douglas

February 24, 2016

A couple years ago, I wrote a book called "Keep on, Keepin' on: A Breast Cancer Survivor Story" about my friend Jean Hanna Davis as she went through her second round of chemotherapy.

Another project I've been working on is titled "Dive-abled: The Leo Morales Story," about a man who lost his entire right leg to cancer and has set world records as a diver.

Cancer has always been a bigger personal issue for me than heart disease. I'm not trying to say that I think cancer is any less important now, of course, but suddenly heart disease prevention has jumped right up there.

Right after coming home from the hospital, a friend referred to me as a survivor. I told my wife that I didn't feel like a survivor, at least not in the same sense as Jean or Leo.

They endured surgery and chemo and radiation and then still had to adapt and change their lives.

In my case, I had two procedures and now I'm adapting my exercise and eating, but all of that is about looking forward and preventing a recurrence.

On the other hand, and something I can't take too lightly, I'm extremely lucky that the blockages in my heart didn't kill me outright. It would have been easy for me to be walking down the street and simply hit the ground.

It didn't occur to me until I was released from the hospital that February is Heart Month. My new-found heart awareness led me to dig into it a little more, and I discovered that we have recognized February as Heart Month longer than I've been alive. President Lyndon Johnson, a heart attack survivor, signed a proclamation declaring it in 1964.

According to the American Heart Association and American Stroke Association, "cardiovascular diseases which include heart disease, stroke, and high blood pressure is the number one killer of women and men in the United States accounting for 17.3 million deaths per year. It is also the leading cause of disability. More than 85 million Americans are living with cardiovascular diseases or the effects of stroke."

It's not like we need to make huge changes to our lives to be more heart-healthy. Get at least 30 minutes of moderate, focused exercise a day, at least five days a week. Eat more fiber and less sodium and saturated and trans fats. It's not like you need to become a vegan or go live in a commune -- unless you want to, of course.

These are simple changes that we can all do.

And maybe with more of us living and not having to deal with heart disease, we can focus our attention on ridding the world of cancer, too.

Lifestyle changes

Since my diagnosis and open-heart surgery, I've made changes to my diet. But let me say right now, I am not perfect. I have lost more than 40 pounds and feel much better. But there are days that I want to eat four or five pieces of candy. Or have a hamburger. Or go to Taco Bell. Or whatever bad behavior comes to mind. I occasionally give in. I feel like denying myself any treats or cheats will just make it worse, or harder to maintain in the long run.

My friend Mac McMillian has an interesting story when it comes to making changes and sticking to them. In 2004, he failed a stress test and a heart catheterization indicated he had blockages. Instead of a surgical intervention, he enrolled in the Dean Ornish program at the local hospital and set to work to reverse his heart disease.

Per the Dr. Dean Ornish website: "Dr. Ornish's Program for Reversing Heart Disease is the first program scientifically proven to 'undo' (reverse) heart disease by optimizing four important areas of your life. This program has been proven to undo heart disease by dealing with the root causes and not just its effects. The combined effect of all four lifestyle elements makes the transformative difference. For more than 35 years, Dean Ornish, MD and his colleagues at the non-profit Preventive Medicine Research Institute (PMRI), have conducted a series of research studies showing that changes in diet and lifestyle can make a powerful difference in our health and well-being, how quickly these changes may occur, and how dynamic these mechanisms can be. Due to better adherence and clinical outcomes than have ever been reported, the Ornish Reversal Program is the first Intensive Cardiac Rehabilitation (ICR) program to be covered by Medicare, as well as national partnerships with many private insurers such as Highmark Inc, Anthem and HMSA."

In the program, Mac went from 330 pounds to 302 pounds, but he couldn't get below 300 pounds. While the Ornish program can be successful, it takes a serious commitment. The program stresses exercise, meditation, yoga, and vegan food preparation. Mac said "I got weary of that grind and slowly eased back into my old habits."

In 2006, Mac ended up having quintuple bypass surgery. "After falling off the Ornish wagon, my health went to shit." Mac was one of those people, though, who didn't make the changes necessary to prolong his life, even after the open-heart surgery.

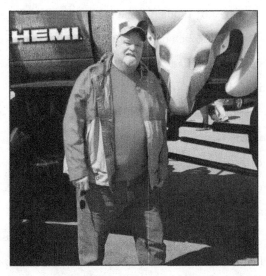

Like a lot of people today, he had a sedentary desk job and ended up putting the weight he lost back on and then climbing higher. Eventually he hit 353 pounds.

Over the next nine years, Mac became severely diabetic and was insulin resistant. He describes the final kick in the head from his friend Steve McCormick. "He said 'Get a damn lapband or you are going to die... soon'."

Mac discussed the surgery with his wife, who happens to be a surgical RN and she suggested his go see Dr. Rossi who performs gastric sleeve surgery. This was in September 2014. It took seven months to get insurance approval for the surgery.

"It's funny, but the sleeve surgery was a bigger kick in the pants than the CABG was," Mac said. "After the sleeve in 2015, I started walking. Then I began the Genesis running program. The interesting thing to me is that heart surgery was a breeze. I don't remember any pain. On the other hand, I saw no immediate change in how I felt. I felt better after sleeve within a week."

Mac's improvements have been tremendous since then. He went from 358 pounds to 224. As of his last blood work a few months ago, all his levels were normal. He still takes a statin and minimum doses of blood pressure medications. He has been off insulin for 18 months.

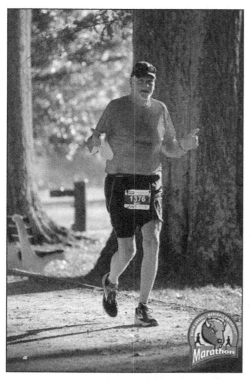

He has also taken up running as more than a hobby or something to do for exercise. It has become a passion for him. He regularly runs in 5 and 10 K races and recently completed a half marathon. He even organized and served as the race director for a 5K race of his own.

"I guess maturity and fear motivates me now to not backslide. You see the world differently after 65 years."

As evidenced by his own experiences, Mac says nothing anyone can say to you will make you change your lifestyle and improve your health.

"You must come to the decision within yourself to want to live longer and happier. Most folks do not believe you can feel better. If your problem is weight-driven, go to a surgical weight loss center and talk to them. Stomach revision surgery is forced portion control, not a magic wand. You, and only you, control WHAT you eat. The surgery just controls HOW MUCH you eat. Weight loss is merely burning more calories than you consume. You must eat a balance that is protein-heavy, and exercise," he explained. "I have become a big supporter of group therapy, too. The weight loss center has monthly free meetings for anyone interested in losing weight."

One of the greatest things I've found to make these changes to my diet and exercise routines is the daily reminder of a fitness tracker on my wrist. Having a daily goal of steps to achieve, and having the tracker on my wrist all the time, made it easier for me to get out of the chair and move.

I had a Fitbit before my surgery, but just after I got home from the hospital, I upgraded to a Fitbit that tracked my heart rate. I did that to keep track of my heart, but it seems to do a better job of keeping track of my calories expended as well.

Changes to diet

For my own journey, I am not on a diet. Or I'm not exercising to get myself in shape. It may sound like a cliché, but this is a lifestyle change. It must be or I am no better off than the people who didn't make the changes in the first place. Maybe I'm worse off like Mac was.

The biggest change for me was cutting down on fast food. As I've said I work from home. I would often plan trips to town for meetings around meals so I could treat myself to a Wendy's hamburger or a Taco Bell run. Those were things I wouldn't fix around the house, so they were special treats for me. Except they weren't. I was probably eating that way two or three times a week.

In my 20s I drank a lot, but that hasn't been an issue for me in a long time. A bigger problem, though, is my sweet tooth. I love candy, and I especially love cookies. I do a lot of cooking and I've always enjoyed baking. For me, especially around the holidays, baking meant family time. It seemed natural to bake cookies or whatever as a treat for my daughters. While those baked treats tasted great, they were full of empty calories and they weren't helping my waistline at all.

I'm a big man. I graduated high school at 6'3" and 205 pounds and was skinny. I graduated college at about 255 and was carrying quite a bit of muscle. That frame allowed me to carry extra weight and for it to not be as noticeable.

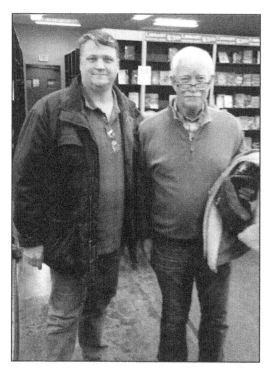

Fully dressed on the day I went in for my stress test, I weighed nearly 300 pounds, (That's me on the left, a week before my stress test, meeting former Marshall University coach Red Dawson) but I remember having a conversation with my cardiologist that I didn't look like I weighed nearly that much. He seemed to think I looked relatively fit. That was why he had doubts about my condition until he got me on the treadmill in his office.

The biggest changes I've made to my diet are adding more fresh vegetables into my daily routine. I eat a salad nearly every day for lunch. It's a big salad, but a pretty good one. I usually add oven-roasted turkey and I've recently replaced cheese on my salad with spiced granola. Sometimes I'll add nuts or trail mix. I try to keep it healthy.

Of course, I have nearly cut out the fast food meals. I'll still have one every occasionally, but it is more like once a month. And then I aim for the chicken sandwiches instead of the double cheese burgers.

Since I do much of the cooking in my house anyway, I can steer our meals toward healthier offerings and no one seems to complain. This includes more baked or grilled chicken, baked fish, and whole grain pasta and bread. We've changed to whole wheat pasta rather than traditional white flour pasta. I honestly don't notice a difference between the two. The texture is a bit different, but it's a small price to pay.

We aren't eating exclusively on a Mediterranean diet, but I try to cook with more olive oil on the rare occasion when I use oil at all. One new dish I've added to our regular menu is what I've named *Pasta a' la Bev*, in honor of my wife. Whole wheat pasta, with mushrooms sautéed in olive oil. Then I add fresh, diced tomatoes, olives and steamed artichokes. Occasionally I throw in grilled chicken or zucchini and squash as well, depending on whatever is fresh at the local farmer's market.

I still eat red meat from time to time, but it is usually in the form of pot roast or a London Broil. That is never more than twice a week and usually less. It is all about balance.

High blood pressure has never been my problem, but I use seasoned salt or other spices to keep my sodium intake down to a minimum. You can add a lot of flavor to food without salt using seasoning mixtures and spices. I found meeting with the nutritionist during cardiac rehab was very helpful. She helped me to understand some of the ways I wasn't helping myself and ways I could improve. As I've said, though, it takes a conscious decision to make these changes. They won't just happen and you can't expect them to stick unless you put them into everyday practice.

The app that comes with my Fitbit allows me to record my food intake, too. It was helpful for me to have my steps, active minutes, calories burned and calories consumed all in one spot. I know there are lots of apps for smartphones that allow you to track exercise and food intake, but this made it very convenient for me. I am not affiliated with Fitbit and I am sure there are others that do a great job, but I have been very pleased with the ease of use and the convenience. It made my recovery that much easier.

Tracking your food intake is a way to learn about your bad habits. Those cookies I like? Often 300 to 500 calories each. A couple of those is equal to an hour on the treadmill at a brisk pace.

One of the biggest keys for me is having a strong support system. My family has been great about not complaining about my healthy food. They've tried my new things and accepted my changes without complaint. (They tell me they like the way I'm cooking now.)

Responses to the Survey

The following is a minimally-edited selection the changes survivors made to their lifestyles. There are very few people in the world who wouldn't benefit from improving their lifestyle, exercise and eating habits. Even fewer of those have some form of coronary artery disease. If you don't make a change following diagnosis and intervention, you are setting yourself up for failure and likely a return to the hospital. Or worse.

There are, of course, a segment of the heart survivors who have low cholesterol and do everything right to begin with. They are very rare. Those people still need to watch their food intake and exercise regularly, too. One survey respondent in an earlier section commented he/she was fit, but not healthy. That is an important distinction to remember. Being fit and exercising regularly doesn't always mean that we are healthy in the way we eat, how we handle stress or when it comes to bad habits like smoking.

Describe the diet and/or exercise changes you made in recovery.

- I became a vegetarian.

- More vegetables, less red meat and cheeses.

- Whole Foods Plant Based Diet (WFPBD) / 30 minutes of walking.

- Vegan diet, exercise at least 1 hour per day.

- I eat all natural foods. For the most part if I could not grow it or raise it, I didn't eat it. I moved for exercise then increased to walking.

- Exercise daily. Clean eating: no sugar, meat or bad fats.

- Less red meat, lowered starches and carbohydrates, lean meats, fruits and veggies and more water!!

- More fruits and veggies and nuts. I drink green tea and hardly any soft drinks.

- No salt or sweet things and daily walk.

- Low salt, low fat diet and walking.

- No fat frying and walk every day.

- Portion control and variety in the diet. Lots of cardiovascular and high intensity workouts.

- Working out 5-days-a-week and trying to follow the Mediterranean diet.

- Walking routine and cutting out sugar and high fat and salt. Still treat myself once a week.

- Switched to a heart healthy diet and walk daily

- Diet: I watch the amount not of red meat I eat and try not to eat as many sweets as I used to. I also eat more fruits and vegetables. Exercise: I work out 4 - 5 times every week for 45 - 1hr periods each time with cardio making up 30-minutes minimum each time.

- I don't follow a certain diet. I just make sure I am eating healthy and following a healthy lifestyle like making sure I get to walk every day and sweat a bit. I also drink loads of water.

- Did 2 months of the Healthy Heart program at the hospital and then joined Curves to continue aerobic exercise. I had been vegetarian for several years before, but now I add some lean poultry, fish and occasionally liver. Substituted good fats for bad and cut down on salt.

- Oatmeal for breakfast often. Less salt and sugar. Less cheese. Try to walk with dog every day for at least a mile.

- I gave up alcohol, fried foods and most veggies due to a blood pressure medication that drives my potassium up, plus I joined a gym.

- Low fat, low sodium and high fiber diet and I do at least 10,000 steps per day.

- Eliminated all processed foods from diet, low sodium diet, try to follow a Mediterranean-style diet and organic/grass-fed meats when possible. Increased amount of exercise. Lots of incline walking on treadmill and small amounts of jogging.

- Cardio rehab. Walking at home. Eating mostly vegetarian. Very aware of cholesterol numbers in food, even though my cholesterol has never been high. Pretty much cut cheeses out. More kale!! More cabbage!!

- I counted calories before, but now I had to cut back and track my sodium and sugar. I'm eating less processed foods and more fruits and veggies. I'm also trying more foods that I wouldn't have tried before. I was sedentary before, but I've just joined a gym after finishing rehab. I'm also walking on my breaks during the day at work.

- Cut out most red meat and all sugar, white bread, rice, etc. Eat a diet rich in vegetables and fruit along with smaller portions. I began to exercise every day and didn't quit. It worked.

- I had never exercised in my life now go to gym three times a week. I was eating lots of chocolate daily, takeout food three times a week and fried unhealthy food. Now I have takeout once a month and one chocolate bar on a Saturday.

- My diet has done a 180. Nothing fried, no sodium, no caffeine. My exercise is still less than what I was doing before.

- I have used the Mediterranean diet as a guide for cooking. I started attending Silver Sneakers classes for strengthening and balance. I walk a couple times a week for additional cardio.

- I try to exercise daily. We have an exercise bike and I watch TV as I peddle. My wife has been cooking healthier.

- Learning to love water and salads. Regular exercising and limiting splurging.

Chapter 9: Rehab

Charleston Gazette-Mail

Learning what I don't know

By Eric Douglas

April 13, 2016

I am self-aware enough to know that I don't know everything, even when I think I do.

When I was at Marshall in the late 1980s, there was a required class called Religious Studies. I watched a lot of freshmen sign up for that class, thinking "Hey, I went to Sunday school. This class will be a breeze."

And they failed it.

They assumed they knew everything, so they didn't apply themselves to it. That lesson has stayed with me for more than 25 years.

For the last month or so, I've been going to cardiac rehab, following up on my open-heart surgery. Exercising in a controlled environment is nothing new for me. I've been doing it most of my life. We had a home weight set with concrete-filled weights when I was a kid. I was about 16 when I joined the local Nautilus and have worked out in, and even worked in, gyms for years.

I really haven't "worked out" all that much in the last few years, however. Work, pressure and other priorities took over and I didn't make time for it. Back "in the day," weightlifting was a much higher priority for me than cardiovascular exercise, anyway.

So, I entered rehab with an open mind and did my best to put my preconceived ideas away.

I'm glad I did. The exercise has been useful and is helping me gain a better understanding of how to push my limits and gain heart strength in the same way I used to push my other muscles. It's also nice to know someone is watching me very closely while I'm pushing it, to make sure I don't push it too far.

The best part of the program though is the education components. I've gained something from nearly every session, probably the most from the discussions about stress management. If you had asked me a few months ago, I would have told you that I really didn't feel stressed. These discussions have opened my eyes to a number of things I've been doing wrong and are helping me change my attitudes so I don't end up back in rehab.

In a lot of ways, I consider myself fortunate to be going through all of this. I could have had a heart attack and never made it to the hospital. Catching my problems when we did has given me the opportunity to make several changes in my lifestyle: eating, stress

management and exercise that will (I hope) keep me
around for a long, long time. There are people
depending on me to be here and I plan to do it for them.

That's probably the most important lesson of all. But
I knew that, already.

Lessons from rehab

Everyone told me that cardiac rehab was the best thing I could do, and I
immediately agreed to sign up for it, but I was still a little nervous when I
showed up for the first day. When I went in for the orientation a few days
earlier, everyone had been upbeat and happy to meet me. They did their
best to put me at ease, of course. But, I knew until I got in there and got to
work, I wouldn't really know how my heart was doing and how I was
healing. My home exercise had gone well, I thought, but you just don't
know. There is a big difference between exercising at home, by yourself,
and doing it in a more public venue with medical professionals watching
you. Had I pushed myself hard enough? Was my heart responding
properly? Would I be able to live an active life again? All those questions
entered my mind at one time or another.

Of course, those were simply self-doubts and had no basis in reality. I
learned about those during one of the information sessions that are part of
rehab: the idea of stamping out ANTs. Those are Automatic Negative
Thoughts. "I can't do that." "It's not doing me any good." "Why do I even
bother?" Those are ANTs. They come to mind whenever things get tough
and you just want to quit.

When I published the newspaper article about starting rehab, a
Facebook friend asked exactly what cardiac rehab was. He had been
through a heart surgery of his own, but his local hospital didn't offer
anything like that. With that in mind, let me explain a little bit more about

what cardiac rehab is, and why all my fears were either baseless or put at ease within moments of beginning the first day.

Cardiac rehabilitation is a combination of monitored exercise and education following heart surgery. I met people who had open-heart surgery, others with stents, valve replacements and other surgeries. I've heard from people who told me they exercised more or less than in my program, but we did four different cardio devices (treadmill, rower, stationary bike, stair climber, etc.) for eight minutes each, with a one minute break in between each one. We exercised wearing three-lead heart monitors so the trained exercise physiologists and nurses could monitor our hearts. They encouraged us to work to a certain level, but slowed us down if our heart rates got too high. The staff took our blood pressure before and after we exercised as well. Participants who were also diabetic had their blood sugar monitored on top of their heart rate.

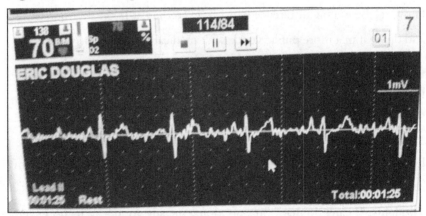

My program also included 20 minute educational programs on topics ranging from stress management and relaxation techniques to diet and the importance of exercise. None of the programs were terribly in-depth, but they weren't supposed to be. They were great introductions to the topics. As part of the rehab program, we also had access to a therapist and a dietitian. The program met for 12 weeks, three days a week. If you missed one, you they just added it onto the end, so you made a total of 36 sessions.

My first day, I was greeted by the class greeter named Tom. Tom was one of three older men named Tom in the group at that time. He started making jokes and talked to everyone as they came in. He was just one of those people. I tried to fill in for him after he graduated.

The interesting thing about the class was that it was a revolving door program. Nearly every week someone graduated or entered the program. The hospital ran five programs every Monday, Wednesday and Friday so there were an awful lot of people being served. They never seemed to run out of patients.

It was rewarding to see others graduate from the program. That meant they had followed through and completed rehab. One of the most disturbing things I heard during the information sessions was that only about 25 percent of people who have had a heart attack or had surgical interventions make changes to their lives. The other 75 percent go home from the hospital and simply wait for it all to happen again. Or to die, I guess.

I met a few people through the class who were repeaters. They had completed rehab, but for whatever reason their heart condition had returned, they had another surgery, and they found themselves going through the process again. I give those people credit, too. It would be exceedingly easy to just quit at that point, but they didn't.

Having a goal when I entered cardiac rehab gave me focus. The staff would always stress that it was important for us to exercise at home. We had to record the amount of time we spent exercising on our own. Most of the time they couldn't believe what I was doing on my own, on top of rehab. On days when I went to rehab, I would often complete another 20 to 30 minutes on the treadmill. One my off days, I would do 40 to 50 minutes of exercise.

For me, cardiac rehab served to benchmark my progress. I could push myself while I was being monitored knowing that the staff would slow me down if they saw any problems. That gave me confidence when I was working out at home.

I will be the first to admit that, in the middle of the program, it turned into a slog. Around the 18th or 20th visit, you start to wonder if it is all worth it or if it is helping. Crossing 30 visits, knowing you have two weeks left, was fantastic. At the end, it was a real sense of accomplishment and I

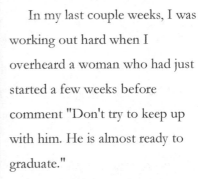

am glad I made it through.

In my last couple weeks, I was working out hard when I overheard a woman who had just started a few weeks before comment "Don't try to keep up with him. He is almost ready to graduate."

By the time I completed my 36th visit to cardiac rehab, I was one of the old hands. Tom had long-since graduated and I had seen a dozen others leave only to be replaced in my 12 weeks. At the graduation, one of the nurses asked if there was anything I wanted to say to the group. I didn't write down what I said, and I really don't remember, but I do know I told the group to set goals for themselves, to push themselves and rely on the staff to have your back. It worked for me.

Responses to the Survey

The following is a minimally-edited selection of comments from survivors about attending a formal cardiac rehab program. Many of the people who attended cite confidence as one of the biggest benefits to the program. The responses are divided between those who went to rehab and those who didn't attend a formal program.

Went

The primary responses in this category were confidence and education.

- Lost 30 pounds, went to two month free (Canada) cardiac rehab. Learned exercise, diet, mental, drugs, etc. Following all advice four years later. Feel great, doing exercises, cardiac & strength in my basement. Heart rate, blood pressure very good (medicated). Very happy to get ahead of my grandpa, dad, younger brother who all had heart attacks and died much younger than I am. Loving life more now.

- I only went for about a month and a half. I just couldn't miss that much work. I didn't enjoy it, but I don't like bike riding and that was really all I could do at the time due to a foot problem.

- A lot of support and it was great to have a steady exercise regimen.

- I got a ton of knowledge on nutrition, exercise, heart rates, and how to best take care of myself.

- Great experience educational and physically and emotionally. I would suggest it for everyone.

- Still involved but it is certainly helping me get my confidence back and notice an improvement during exercise.

- It helped me be confident again. To trust my body again.

- It helped develop an exercise regimen.

- Strengthening of my heart and confidence in myself.

- Excellent education. I have to constantly renew what I learned though.

- Confidence builder as I could do a lot more than the rehab required of me.

- Attending rehab gave me the outlet to get active again. Due to my cycling background, it was a breeze and cleared me to ride on the road once again.

- Enjoyed it. Carrying it on at my local gym.

- Great, like having a personal trainer for a few weeks after surgery.

- I learned that it was safe to exercise. I got nutrition information. I was the youngest one in the group.

- Learned to build myself up a little bit at a time.

- Really all I got out of it was being with people that understood.

- Still haven't completed the program due to latest event. I've never been much of an exerciser (active, but no gym rat). Really enjoyed the support of others who have been there. And the safe feeling of initially exercising while being monitored.

- It made me stronger & more confident in not only exercising but even doing everyday things. I didn't feel strong after surgery, but rehab made me realize that not only was I not broken but I was a warrior now. It was the best choice I could have made, even if I was the youngest one there. The comradery between the patients helped a lot in the mental recovery, too.

- Cardiac Rehab got me on my feet. I was weak after surgery and it helped a lot.

- A ton! I loved it. It was inspiring, although I was the only one under 75. It was educational & they helped me a lot.

- I got physically stronger and confident that I could resume activities without endangering my heart.

- It was the best program ever. I practically crawled to my first rehab class, I was so weak. But this class helped me to get my strength back and my confidence to do things again.

- Tons and it continues. He works on getting stronger

- It was huge in my mental and physical recovery. I totally embraced it.

Didn't go

Several people in this category said they were not told about the program, it wasn't offered, or their insurance didn't cover it. Those answers are all a shame. Others said they didn't think they would get much out of it.

- My little dog went blind and diabetic. She suffered extreme separation anxiety. I decided to do my own rehab at home.

- 100 miles from town...executed my own rehab at home, walking and riding a bike.

- Insurance didn't cover.

- Wasn't offered. Diagnosis was reflux and recommended lifestyle changes.

- Doctor never discussed it. I only heard about it on heart attack survivor's website, but by then it had been two years after my heart attack.

- I had no insurance.

- Because I went back to work after a month and cardiac rehab is offered on weekdays only.

- My doctor never mentioned it to me. Being new to the world of heart disease, it's not something I knew was available to me.

- There was no rehabilitation program at that hospital.

- I began and participated a couple of times. But, I had to get back to work, I had no choice.

- No because I wanted to work out in a gym my own way, also didn't want to hear any horror stories from others.

- Too expensive for me since it was 100% out of pocket.

- Had my own plan, advised by doctor.

Chapter 10: Recovered

Charleston Gazette-Mail

Coming full circle, underwater

By Eric Douglas

August 24, 2016

For nearly 20 years, I've made a career in scuba diving. It has taken me all over the world and away from West Virginia for 14 years, first to California and then to North Carolina. Since I've been back, I still write about diving regularly for Scuba Diving Magazine, as well as in my adventure novels.

You can probably see why getting back under the water was so important to me following my open-heart surgery. I don't dive nearly as much as I used to, but the idea that I couldn't dive at all was all the motivation I needed to get to work.

My first 60-plus scuba dives were in Summersville Lake before I ever made a dive in the ocean. Once I got permission to dive again from my doctor, I debated running down to Florida to go diving with friends, but I realized I needed to go back to my roots; back to the beginning, as it were.

Life had come full circle for me and that meant I needed to make my first dive in my second chance at life in Summersville Lake. And there was only one dive buddy I wanted beside me on that trip: my dad.

I moved to Southern California in 1998 to take a job in scuba diving. About that time, my dad (Ralph Douglas) decided he wanted to learn to dive, too. A year or so later, he came to visit in California and we made our first dives together. It was a really cool experience. Since then we've dived together in North Carolina and here many times.

About a week after my birthday and just a few days before my dad's 78th birthday, we took a day and ran up to Summersville. Conditions on the lake were good and the weather was relatively mild. I probably should have been a little nervous to dive again, all things considered, but it really didn't go through my mind. I simply wanted to feel weightless again. And I wanted to get that monkey off my back.

I often tell my daughters that they have to have a plan when they start something or they will never finish it. I guess I lived out my own lesson.

And I got to go diving at the same time.

Return to diving

While I was waiting for my date with the surgeon I committed to myself that I was going to return to scuba diving status. While you don't have to be a super-human swimmer or anything like that, you do have to have a good level of fitness. Most of the time diving is a relaxed sport. Divers are taught to swim slowly and easily. Water resistance makes it harder to move quickly and all that does is make you tired and out of breath without really accomplishing much. On the other hand, as a diver you must be fit enough

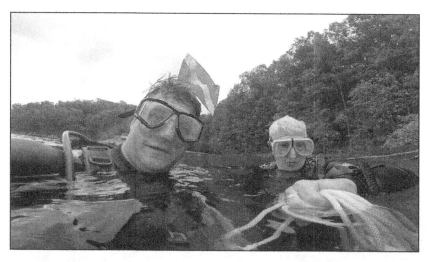

to respond to an emergency and swim hard and fast if necessary.

I knew all of that before my surgery. To be honest, I've known it for years and even answered other people's questions about it when I was asked. So, when I was told I was scheduled for open-heart surgery, I knew it was possible to return to diving, but I also knew it would take a lot of hard work to get there.

You see, divers are expected to demonstrate a basic level of fitness when they are certified initially, but (at least in the United States) they never have to do it again. You perform basic swim tests and then there is no recertification. It is assumed that divers without known heart disease are fit enough to dive. Groups like the British Sub Aqua Club require regular diving physicals.

Having open-heart surgery doesn't disqualify you from ever diving again, but you do have to achieve a higher level of fitness than the average diver before being cleared to dive again. The water pressure and the physical effort of swimming and breathing through a regulator at depth increases the work load on your heart. Additionally, the remote locations (even just out on dive boats) make having another cardiac event more deadly. EMS response is almost impossible and you rely on bystander CPR from the boat crew or passengers.

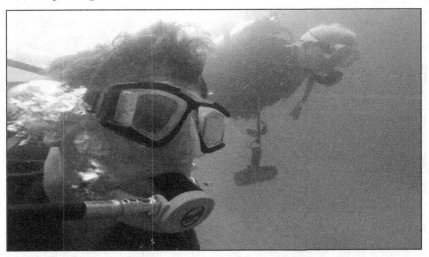

Once you have to check off that you have had a heart attack or coronary artery disease or open-heart surgery on a diving release form, you have to have your doctor's permission. In the medical community, the gold standard is that you can perform exercise to 13 METs. A MET is a metabolic equivalent and one MET is amount of energy burned by a person seated at rest. Achieving 13 METS requires jogging at 4.2 miles per hour at a 16 percent grade (after working through the previous stages) for about a minute. This is Stage 4 of the Bruce Protocol.

It may seem unfair that a diver with no history of heart disease should have no performance requirements while one with a history must exercise to that level, but a doctor told me they would much prefer all divers could demonstrate 13 METS, but they can't enforce that. They can with those with a known history.

As I've said, I've never been a runner. I liked to bike and swim, but jogging or running were never high on my list. In the months leading up to my heart diagnosis, I had become even less interested in aerobic activity. So, when I got home from the hospital, it was all I could do to take two six minute walks at 1.5 miles an hour with no incline.

Still, that was my baseline. I knew where I had to be and I got to work. I kept that goal in my mind every day and kept pushing. Just a little bit faster, or a little bit farther every day. While there was no real reason for it, I decided I wanted to get back to diving status by my 49th birthday. That would be almost exactly six months after my surgery.

Of course, there were setbacks and bad weeks along the way. But ultimately, I made it. I got cleared to dive by my cardiologist and my surgeon a couple weeks before my birthday in July. I didn't make it underwater until a week or so after my birthday, but it was close enough.

The most important part of the process, and my recovery, was having a goal. I focused on that and pushed toward it every day. Just saying "I want to get healthy" or "I want to get in shape" would not have cut it for me. I had to have a definite, measurable goal with a specific timetable. If it took me eight months instead of six, I think that would have been fine. I might have gotten discouraged when I missed the deadline, but the next day I would have gotten back on the treadmill and focused that much more.

Ultimately, my advice to anyone recovering from a diagnosis like this, or trying to achieve anything difficult, really, is to have a specific goal. I tell my teenage daughters this on a regular basis. Saying "I want to do..." won't make anything happen. As the French writer Antoine de Saint-Exupery said, "A goal without a plan is just a wish."

Set a measurable goal and work toward it every day. It should be an achievable goal, but one that makes you stretch a little bit. As I said, I was never a runner. This wasn't a situation where I would be returning to my previous running form. I had to start from scratch. But I did it.

It won't happen overnight, but you will get there.

Responses to the Survey

The following is a minimally-edited selection of comments from survivors about completing their recovery. A number of respondents said it wasn't complete yet. Whether that meant they were still early in the process, or that they felt their recovery would never be complete and would always have to work at it, we don't know.

What did you achieve that made you feel your recovery was complete?

- I can walk at least two miles or more now.
- Went back to work.
- Changed to a whole-foods plant-based diet and was off statins and blood thinners in 90 days with a total cholesterol of 107 after 10 months without statins.
- Successfully being able to run my normal day without shortness of breath or fatigue.
- Back to normal life and even better - I had to be back on the court.
- Back to work, albeit part time in the beginning, and increasing to full time. Gave me a sense of routine again.
- Didn't live with constant anxiety anymore. My follow up appointment showed recovery.
- Lost the weight temporarily and felt better.
- Still working on full recovery, but a main goal will to be off some meds in less than two years.

- My recovery will never be complete; it is ongoing. A big step for me was being able to ride my horse.

- Chest soreness disappearing, blood pressure better, losing weight and feeling better.

- Training with a coach for a triathlon next year.

- I achieved the ability to not only do day-to-day activity without running out of breath but also to do long bicycle rides.

- Back to the day-to-day activities and feeling good.

- Felt better about life and went back to work at five months.

- Lost 29 pounds and felt "normal" with activity.

- Able to lift reasonable amount of weight, run with the dog, forgetting for several hours at a time that I had had open-heart surgery.

- I suppose I would say I still struggle, but I am so grateful to be alive I want to keep things in perspective. Realizing how blessed I am to be alive.

- I stopped taking my anxiety meds and have accepted the new me.

- I became able to work my job and do household chores again.

- I was told that most of the muscle damage on the back of my heart had healed, and my ejection fraction is at 65%.

- It's never complete. My life is entirely different from my precardiac experience.

- I gained control of my life. I also realized that so many things contributing to my problem are hereditary so I make sure I take all my medication religiously and keep all doctors appointments every 6 months.

- 200 press ups a day 7 days a week

- Ride my mountain bike, although I know I will never be at where I was.

- Being able to drive again and then going back to work.

- Proper exercise and strength returned.

- I'm not there yet, but I think it will be when I don't feel as tired and don't have as much chest muscle pains. It'll be lovely to sleep on my side without a problem again, too!

- I could exercise strongly. I didn't tire at all during the day. I was pain free and I feel great.

- I did the race for life for cancer!! Something I had never done before!! I was back to work and pretty much back to how I was before it all happened.

- I was able to go grocery shopping without needing a motorized scooter.

- I am able to do almost everything that I did before the heart attack. I recently took a trip that involved a six-hour drive. I can do three loads of laundry, climbing the steps from the basement and to the second-floor multiple times in a day.

- More self confidence in doing activities and traveling some.

- I lost weight, brought my sugar down and eating healthier, thanks to the wife.

- Skateboarding full on, building sculptures at my normal pace, working all day in the studio and not feeling dizzy spells.

- Ability to resume activities of daily living, including taking my son to school, going to the mall by myself, and ordering my own lunch.

Chapter 11: Psychological Stress

The changes that come with heart disease and the aftermath of an intervention (surgery, stents, rehab) aren't all physical. I've talked to many survivors who struggled with the loss of physical ability and the emotional/psychological changes that come with it.

Honestly, I don't recall ever being depressed after my surgery. Frustrated? Sure. But I never got into the tailspin that I've heard so many people describe. I can only attribute that to having a goal and a plan. Before I left the hospital, I knew what I had to do. I got frustrated about how slow it was moving or my inability to meet my possibly unrealistic goals, but I never felt like I wouldn't be able to achieve what I wanted to do.

A second bonus for me was just a few days after I came home from the hospital, I returned to work. At least a little. I went (slowly) downstairs and sat at my computer for a while. I fully understand most people don't have this opportunity.

The problem I faced was my attention span was significantly shorter. Whether it was from being tired or in discomfort or the healing process, I don't know, but it made it harder to focus on something long enough to write for any length of time. I could write a 400-word newspaper column about my heart recovery, but to sit down and work on an 85,000-word novel was impossible. I couldn't even write 500 words in a project like that, because I couldn't focus well enough to keep the story straight in my mind.

In fact, I was working on a novel when I went into the hospital and I had to put it aside. It took me nine months to pick that project back up again.

For most people, your identity is tied up in the work that you do. It is how you contribute to the world and care for your family. After surgery, you have to accept that other people have to do most of what you are used to doing for yourself. And you start worrying about how you are going to provide for your family.

In my case, as a freelancer and writer, I had those same thoughts, of course. While I got to work immediately, the fear was still there. I don't have sick leave. If I'm not producing, no one is paying me. So I felt the need to do work immediately. I couldn't convalesce and rest. It was a two-edged sword.

As I said, I didn't feel depressed, but I do remember being more agitated and angry. Or at least quicker to anger. I would snap at the smallest of slights or create issues in my head that didn't exist for anyone but me.

Looking back, I can attribute that to a lot of things. I wasn't sleeping well. I would get a few hours of sleep in the bed and have to move to my recliner to finish the night. I was tired because my body was trying to recover. I was in pain. It wasn't excruciating, but it was nearly constant. (That was a big part of the reason I wasn't sleeping.) I'm sure there was also a certain amount of anxiety in there, too.

I still remember one evening, a few weeks after surgery, when my daughters came to spend the weekend. It was the first time I'd gotten to spend any time with them since I got home from the hospital. They got into a fight about something and I just lost it. I ended up screaming at both of them. Still today, the memory of that evening upsets me. I apologized to them later, but I know they were both afraid of me for a while afterward.

That hurts me more than the surgery ever could have.

We all know the term Post Traumatic Stress Disorder when it comes to veterans or first responders who have trouble adjusting to daily life after the stressful situations of combat or a particularly grisly or disturbing accident scene (just to name a few situations.)

It had never occurred to me that I was struggling with a form of PTSD myself until I read through the comments of several survey respondents who mentioned it. Several survey respondents also talked about anxiety throughout their recovery. Doing some research, I found several scholarly articles that indicated that heart and stroke survivors are at risk of PTSD after a cardiac event and that "PTSD should not be ignored as a sequel of heart disease, given preliminary evidence that PTSD may be associated with nonadherence with medication and an increased risk of clinical adverse events." [2]

In my case, the anxiety, or PTSD, was short-lived and I have returned to my normal outlook on life. The important thing to remember while you are recovering from surgery is to give yourself time to heal. It will not go perfectly. The psychological part of recovery is just as important as the physical side. My cardiac rehab program offered visits with a psychologist as part of the program. I think that is an important part of healing.

A lot of people, mostly men, will never take advantage of the ability to talk to a professional. If you don't do that, at least talk to your spouse or a close friend. You can't keep those feelings bottled up inside of you. I will admit I never spoke to the psychologist. I never felt a need for it. After the incident with my daughters, I realized I was much more agitated and did my best to identify those feelings and recognize them for what they were. I tried to be aware of unusual feelings and think through them before I let them grow to another outburst.

I had several conversations with my wife where we talked about how close I came to dying and the mistakes I made leading up to the surgery by denying the symptoms I was experiencing. We talked about goals and the future, too.

There is no one way to get through this. The keys to recovery, for me, are to have a goal, to be active and to talk to others about how you are feeling. Don't hold it all in.

Responses to the Survey

The following is a minimally-edited selection of comments from survivors about their strength level after the recovery process. There are cases where damage to the heart muscle itself will make returning to full strength nearly impossible. The comments are divided into three categories: Not as Strong As, As Strong As and Stronger Than Before.

Why do you feel you are not as strong, or stronger than, before your recovery?

Not as Strong

- Just feel like I don't have near the stamina for anything I once had.
- It is physically apparent when I try to accomplish things I was able to do prior to surgery.
- An ejection fraction of 35 limits some of things I can do.
- I am unable to maintain heavy work as I did before. Medication seems to bring on more bruising and chances for injury in my line of work with horses.
- I think I am not as strong because the damage to my heart to irreversible. All I can do is prevent from anymore of my heart being damaged.

- Two other blockages that are not stented. I can feel my heart is not as strong.

- I still lack the energy to be doing has much as I should be.

- I wasn't told this at the time of my event, but my daughter was told I would most likely have motor skill and memory problems due to coding for so long. My short-term memory isn't as good as it used to be, but I go to work each day and work on complex government regulations, and live my life all by myself. I do have early onset osteoarthritis as well, and was told that in my case the aging process has sped up a bit. I also struggle with chronic pain like fibromyalgia - this is also new. I used to lift weights in the gym 3-4 times a week, and now I am just tired a lot. It's a deep sense of loss for me.

- Just don't have the stamina that I used to have and now I have trouble sleeping.

- Because I'm not. Prior to the heart attack, I was in the gym lifting heavy weight. I haven't tried, but I know I'm not close to being as strong. Just bringing in the groceries, I can't carry near as much before.

- My weight is way down and have less muscle mass. At 6' tall, formerly 200 lbs., currently 167 lbs.

- Fear of having another heart attack so I limit any exertions.

- I still suffer from shortness of breath, fatigue and weakness.

- Heart badly damaged so muscle weakness and exhaustion is a normal thing now.

- I have to get 9-10 hours asleep a night and I used to get 4! I don't get as much done as I used to and I just had to get used to it. That took a while.

- The Thelemic stroke left him with pain and mobility issues. Mentally, he struggles with forced retirement and losing his ability to fly as well.

As Strong as Before

- I am very healthy, I can breathe, and walk long distances without losing my breath. I can play with my granddaughter, get in her little ball pit and not be uncomfortable.
- I feel that there is no change in my strength from before quintuple bypass. Now that I am back to my job (physical) I can perform all the tasks that I did before.
- I have detailed records of all my training going back six years. There is no noticeable change.
- I feel stronger than when I received my fourth diagnosis and recovery. Though I cannot cycle like I did 12 years ago, nor at the level of a lot of other 66-year old cyclists.

Stronger Than Before

- I feel I like I am much stronger.
- I feel better than before surgery.
- Gained a lot of weight, but quitting smoking makes me stronger.
- I can run/elliptical for 30+ minutes every day.
- Better wind, longer, faster walks, etc.
- Work out every day, have endurance I haven't had in years.
- At one year, I was being more active than before the heart attack.
- Nothing holds me back. I push forward every day and do the best I can every day.
- In much better physical condition. I lost 30 pounds and have

better tolerance for exercise.

- I was forced to be strong when I didn't know I could be that strong. I would have never thought I could undergo such a brutal surgery and not only survive, but come out so much more mentally stronger. I truly hope to become more of an advocate with the American Heart Association and am honored to be a feature story for a local event in May for their Go Red for Women event.

- I feel wonderful. I know that prior to the surgery I didn't and just wasn't aware of how I felt.

- I feel that I have a fresh start and life is not forever.

- My body is working well. I am happy and living a great life for 13 years now.

Chapter 12: Moving Forward

Charleston Gazette-Mail
Team Second Chance
By Eric Douglas
July 27, 2016

Today is my 49th birthday.

I'm not telling you that to get attention. Realistically, my mom did all the work this day 49 years ago, so thank you, Mom!

I bring up my birthday because, six months ago, I was in the hospital waiting on open-heart surgery.

I had absolute faith in Dr. Figueroa and wasn't worried about the surgery itself. What I realized then is a little more than a week before that I had been shoveling snow. A month before that, I had a heart attack that I denied.

If things had gone differently, I might never have made it to the hospital for that surgery. From there, I never would have gotten the chance to celebrate this birthday.

A few days after my surgery, while I was recovering in the hospital, my youngest daughter, Jamison, told me that some people regard times like this as a new birthday. It's a chance to restart and look at everything with a new eye.

When I got home from the hospital, my friend, Danny Boyd, welcomed me to the Second Chance Club.

I liked where both of them were headed. I was given another shot and I'm not about to waste it.

Before I left the hospital, I determined I was going to get in shape to be given permission to scuba dive again. I got that letter signed a couple weeks ago. I haven't been diving yet, but I will soon.

That goal met, it's time to shift gears and set my sights on a new one. Without something to shoot for, it would be too easy for me to backslide and lose the gains I've made.

My next target is to jog a 5K race. Not just walk it, but I want to jog the 3.1 miles at a decent pace.

That said, I don't really care if I am the last one to finish. This is about me pushing myself, not competing with others.

The Charleston Heart Walk is Sept. 10. I've set up a team on the Charleston Heart Walk website, called Team Second Chance and hope to get some friends to join me. (You don't have to jog with me, if you don't want. Just come out and walk.) You can search by team names to join me.

My goal is to give more people a second chance at life and hopefully spare some of those people the pain of open-heart surgery. Maybe we'll all celebrate a few more birthdays, as well. We'll call your participation a birthday present to both of us.

#

Once I was cleared to dive again by my doctors, it was almost anticlimactic to actually go diving. Just the feeling of being told I could dive again was almost enough.

After I went diving, I knew I needed to set a new goal. If I didn't have something to work for, I would begin to backslide. Part of my training goal as I worked my way back to diving status was to be able to jog three miles without stopping. That was where I found my next goal. I wanted to run a 5K race.

"Run" is a bit of a misnomer, though. I wanted to jog or shuffle my way through 3.1 miles and complete a 5K at faster than a walking pace. I had no delusions about speed or finishing times. It worked out perfectly that the West Virginia chapter of the American Heart Association was holding their Heart Walk fundraiser in Charleston on September 10, 2016. The heart walk is a 5K, but it wasn't a timed 5K. It is a walk and fun run. That was perfect or me. I wouldn't feel any pressure to compete or meet a time. I could trot my way through the distance and complete the race.

When I decided to do the heart walk, I had never actually completed jogging three miles. Probably the best I could do was two miles. I didn't actually make a full three miles on my home treadmill until a week before the Heart Walk.

Since I had been so public about my recovery, I wanted to keep that up and to use it as leverage to get some other people involved. I set up a team on the Heart Walk page and started asking people to join me and started asking for donations.

When race day arrived, there were five of us on the team, but we had raised $500 for the American Heart Association. That put Team Second Chance in the top five of the non-corporate teams. Many thanks to Lera

VanMeter, Paul and Raveena Saluja and Todd Reynolds for coming out and supporting me. Todd ran alongside me as well and kept me going for the whole 5K.

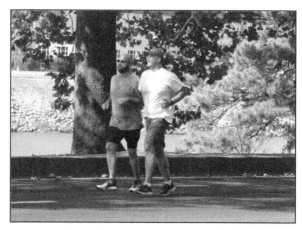

Completing that goal and hurdle felt really good.

Since then, I almost never jog for a distance shorter than three miles and typically go three and a half miles. I'm working on going faster bit by bit as well.

Responses to the Survey

The following is a minimally-edited selection of comments from survivors about the goals they set as part of their own recovery. Most said lose weight or stop smoking and to improve fitness.

What was your health or fitness goal?

- To get back to running and walking at least five miles a night.
- To be able to work out without fear.
- To walk 30 minutes with getting winded.
- Exercise every day for 45 minutes to an hour
- Maintain healthy blood pressure for 40 minutes of exercise.
- To walk around our block (2.5 km) without being tired.
- Walking briskly daily and getting back to 40 hr. work week.
- Lose 100 pounds and be active instead of sedentary.

- I want to live and spend time with my grandchildren. I was able to go back to work and able to ride my horse.

- Initially the London to Brighton bike ride nonstop, accomplished 8 months post op. New goal is Ironman Barcelona 70.3 May 2017.

- To walk every day increasing distance. To go back to the gym 3X/week. To eat healthier.

- To be able to exercise on elliptical for 40min straight. Lose some weight.

- I went back to work at 10 weeks and slowly went back to walking about a mile each day.

- I began walking. At first I could only walk a few feet. In a month or so I was up to 4 miles a day.

- For the past 18 months, I've attended the gym three times a week and for the past three months, five times a week for two hours. One hour cardio.

- Originally lose 50 pounds, I'm at 90.

- Be able to sing and walk up my driveway.

- I wanted to change my eating & exercising habits to allow myself to live a long (& heart attack free) life. I did drastically change my eating habits.

- Fitness. I wanted to be strong enough to be able to continue to live independently in my three-story house. That means going up stairs frequently, doing chores that involve carrying things like clothes baskets, cat litter, and trash, as well as walking for shopping and fun. I wanted to be able to travel as I had been doing to take art classes in New Mexico and other places.

- My hope was to reach a point where I could start cycling on a regular basis.

- Get back to previous physical condition. The goals set by therapists kept me going.
- To get back on the ski slopes in 2017. I was already quite fit as a lifelong skateboarder...but I missed skiing this past year. I did not need to lose weight or change diet much, but I did lose a few pounds in the process.

Chapter 13: Final Thoughts

Charleston Gazette-Mail

When one door closes ...

By Eric Douglas

June 1, 2016

This week, I've completed my cardiac rehab and I feel ready for the next phase of my life.

As a reminder, in January, I failed a stress test miserably and bought myself a stay at CAMC Memorial for open-heart surgery to repair five coronary artery blockages.

It was a scary, frightening time. But even before I got out of the hospital, I knew I was going to write about the process. My first column, written from my hospital bed and published the day I was released from the hospital (to the amusement of my surgeon), was "Don't Make the Same Mistakes I Did."

My hope in writing about my recovery is that some of you might read my story and make some changes in your own lives -- or at least go see your doctor. (A number of people have written to me to tell me that they did just that.) I also thought some of you might read my story and have a better understanding of what would happen if you got the same diagnosis I did, making the process not so scary.

A few people have asked me if I feel better than I ever have before. I doubt I will ever feel as good as I did in my 20s, so that's not going to happen, but I can safely say that I feel better now than I did before I went into the hospital and probably better than I've felt in at least a year. It's amazing how we can accept slight decreases in our health, justifying them away without realizing there was an underlying cause.

Now that I am done with cardiac rehab, I'm not about to slow down. I'm planning to diversify my home exercise some more, adding in some more swimming and biking, but I am not about to slack off. Any time I think I don't feel like exercising or if I want to eat something I shouldn't, I just rub the scar in the center of my chest and I get motivated and back on track. My goal is to be able to return to scuba diving status in the very near future.

I have to send out a big thanks to everyone who took care of me, from my cardiologist to the hospital staff and then everyone at cardiac rehab at Charleston Area Medical Center (CAMC)— Memorial. You've put me on the right track and I won't let you down.

#

Overall, I think I've done pretty well, maintaining my diet and exercise routines. Pretty well isn't perfect, though. But I don't think that's a bad thing.

I said it before, but I don't think of the changes I've made to my diet as being on a diet. It's a lifestyle change. It must. When people go on a diet, they expect it to end and then return to their previous eating habits. I know I can't do that, not if I want to stay out of the hospital and healthy.

At the same time, if I beat myself up or got discouraged when I had a package of M and Ms or indulged in a cheese burger, it would be easy to just give up and quit. Ultimately, I let myself have something that doesn't exactly go with a heart-healthy diet from time to time. I know I do well most of the time and that is enough. This is a marathon, not a sprint. In the same way that I can't expect to fix everything wrong with me in a few weeks or months, I can't let a small blip derail me, either.

After completing the Heart Walk 5K, I will be the first to admit that I got off track a bit. I didn't have a new goal to push myself toward. I was still exercising, but I eased up on my diet a bit. I was happy with my weight so I decided I would go into a maintenance mode.

And that's when the curve ball hit me. I do most of my aerobic exercise on a home treadmill. It's a little under two years old, so it is still under warranty, which is a good thing. One day as I was jogging along, it just stopped. Attempts to reset it didn't work. I won't bore you with the details, but it ultimately took three tries and about a month and a half to get it fixed and working again.

Fortunately, it was fall and the weather was nice. I was able to exercise outside most of the time I wanted. My neighborhood is hilly, though, and it started taking a toll on my knees. As the pain increased, it was harder to force myself to go outside and run. I started slacking off.

About the same time, we came upon Halloween and suddenly there was candy in the house. I've had a sweet tooth since I was a kid and it is hard for me to resist.

My overall weight didn't go up much, just a couple pounds, but I just didn't feel as good as I had. With exercise and achievement comes a feeling of euphoria and that was gone. Losing that, though, makes it even harder to get motivated to exercising. I'm sure there is a psychological term for this, but I'll just call it a downward spiral.

The final straw came when I had a business trip. I knew it was going to be difficult to eat right on the trip so I resolved I wasn't going to stress about it too much. I would control what I could and then forgive myself.

What helped kick me back into gear consisted of three things. On the business trip, I ran into several friends and associates I hadn't seen since before my surgery. Since I had been so public about it, through the convenience of social media, they all knew what I had gone through. So many people came up and wished me well or told me how good I looked and that I looked "healthy." It was very inspiring and had me resolving to get back on the stick as soon as I got home.

The second thing that got me moving was setting another goal just before I left on the trip. My first 5K run was really a fun run in support of the American Heart Association. It wasn't a timed 5K. Just before I left on my trip, I decided to sign up for an official, timed 5K race. While I had no aspirations of winning or anything like that, I knew the idea of running with people who were pushing their speeds would make me run harder, too. As soon as I got home, I knew I had to get back to training and do a better job of watching my diet again. No more slacking.

The third thing that got me back on the right track was getting my treadmill fixed finally. A lot of people hate running on a treadmill, but for me it helps me stay focused. It is so much easier for me to work for a while in the morning and then go into the next room, jog for 45 minutes, cool off, take a shower and get back to work. I don't have to get dressed, or jump in the car and go somewhere.

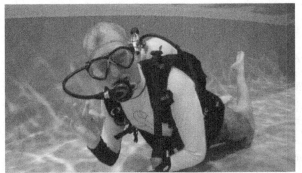

Another bit of inspiration during this period of backsliding was my friend Greg, the radio show host, hit the three-month mark in his recovery. He wasn't cleared to make a full scuba dive of his own, but to celebrate his own return to health, he planned to make a dive in a four-foot deep pool at a conference we were both attending. He invited his friends to join him in and out of the water. It was great to see the smile on Greg's face underwater (I was behind the camera) and on the surface. He had crossed that hurdle and proven to everyone around that you can come back from open-heart surgery to do whatever you want to do.

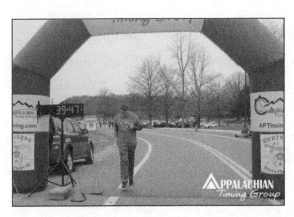

When I got home from the conference, I started training in earnest and a couple weeks later, I participated in the Snowflake 5K, sponsored by the Shriners Beni Kedem Temple as a fundraiser (organized by Mac MacMillian that you met earlier). The course was mostly flat, but right in the middle of the course is a long, steep hill. I planned to run the 5K in under 40 minutes. On the treadmill, I could do 5K in 37 minutes, but I knew that hill would slow me down. I finished it in 39:32.5. I was very pleased with my final result. It turned out that I was last place in my age group, but that didn't matter. Out of 162 participants, I was 75th place overall so it wasn't like I finished last, either.

In general, I am not a competitive person. I don't feel the need to beat everyone around me. On the other hand, I do push myself. I want to better myself and continue to improve. Moving forward into my second year in my second chance life, I see the need to maintain some sort of goal. I do not expect to start training for a marathon or anything like that, but I see the need to have fitness goals. Simply maintaining what I have isn't going to cut it. I can see how that attitude got me out of my routine

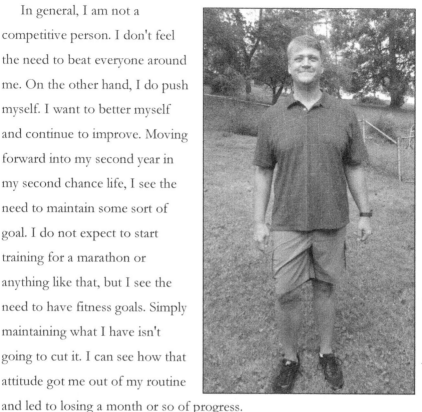

and led to losing a month or so of progress.

In a lot of ways, I feel as if my recovery is over. My health is better than it has been in years. The doctors are happy with me and I like the way I look and feel. But that doesn't mean I get to slack off, either. This isn't a diet. I have to continue with my new lifestyle so I can continue with my life.

Lessons

There are lots of lessons we can learn as heart and stroke survivors. For me, before everything else, it is to remember that recovery is a marathon, not a sprint. Many survivors never feel as if they are fully recovered. Ultimately, I believe they are right. This isn't something you can do for a few months, or even a year, and then go back to living the way you did before your diagnosis, heart or stroke event, and surgery. You have to change the very way you've been living.

Some people will say they can't do it. I get that. It feels like it is unfair, or you are being punished. I don't know that we were ever promised "fair" to begin with, but that is an entirely different subject. If you aren't willing to make the required changes to improve your health, you will never get better and no amount of wishing will change that. Even if you do make those changes, there is no guarantee that you will get "better." I believe it beats the alternative, however.

I receive regular emails from the marketing guru Seth Godin. Sometimes they are marketing specific, and other times they speak to our overall mindset. One recently spoke to me with regards to this issue. It said.

"Entitlement is optional.

"It's not forced on us, it's something we choose.

"And we rarely benefit from that choice.

"That emergency surgery, the one that saved your life, when the ruptured appendix was removed—the doctor left a scar.

"We can choose to be grateful for our next breath.

"Or we can find a way to be enraged, to point out that given how much it costs and how much training the doctor had, that scar really ought to be a lot smaller. And on top of that, he wasn't very nice. We're entitled to a nice doctor!

"Or we can choose to be grateful."

I did everything wrong. I was overweight and I wasn't exercising. I ate the wrong foods. And it caught up with me. I denied it, and rationalized it, when the signs were right in front of my face that something was wrong. I believed I needed to be strong for my family. And I could have died.

My road to recovery hasn't been perfect and it hasn't been straight. I am awed by the people I have heard from who made dramatic, nearly instant changes in their lives. They became vegetarians. They immediately started exercise routines and haven't wavered. Most of us don't fall into that category.

The thing that helped me the most was that I had a concrete goal. I wanted to return to scuba diving. I knew what I would need to do and I set out to achieve it. Even on the days that I slacked off, or ate what I wasn't supposed to eat, I still had that goal hanging in front of me. It gave me focus and it drove me forward.

The second most important thing, or maybe 1A, was a strong support system. I was heartbroken reading through some of the comments from survivors who said they didn't have support, or their kids and friends were "worthless." I can't imagine facing any of this without support. On the other hand, I was impressed by how many people said they found strength and inspiration in the form of online or Facebook support groups. Whatever it takes to motivate you and keep you working is exactly what you need. There is no right or wrong. If you aren't getting support at home, then online is the next best thing.

I get frustrated when I hear things like the statistic that only 25 percent of survivors make permanent changes to their lives. When you are given a second chance at life, why would you squander it? The last thing in the world I want to go through is open-heart surgery for a second time. I will do whatever I can to avoid that. Ultimately, we just have to keep fighting.

As survivors, we have been given a second (or third) chance. Let's not blow it.

I choose to be grateful for every day I have.

Responses to the Survey

Please write any additional stories you would like to share related to your recovery and rehabilitation that I haven't asked about.

- I sometimes struggle with memory. I believe they call this pumphead syndrome. I have an extremely mild case of it compared to others I have read about. I wish maybe this would be explained a little in cardiac rehab. If only so I didn't think I was losing my mind.

- As a result of my heart attack, I was terminated from my nonprofit job of eight years after attending cardiac rehab 3x per week for 12 weeks. I had to rebuild most of my professional life from the ground up in one year. Family tends to not understand the emotional effects and depression that results from these events. I believe there should be more information available to those under 55 who have suffered and survived major events. Our lives are forever changed!

- In ICU, I could only walk 10 steps and I was already tired. I am a positive person and to get better fast also depended on my state of mind.

- The heart is amazing where my collateral arteries actually made its own bypass to save me from severe heart damage. I believe I have less than 5% heart damage and b/c of this and my EF is 55%. I was very lucky as all heart attack survivors and plan to do the best to make my second chance as worthwhile as possible. Lastly, you have to be your own health advocate and ask many questions of your doctors until you are satisfied with their answers. They are very busy and will push you off if they think you are doing fine and you are one less person for them to worry about and/or treat.

- Anxiety and depression is real. It can mimic heart symptoms from pain to blood pressure.

- I believe people have to pay attention to symptoms both medical and nutritional. Freda and I have had a nutritional web site since 1997 and I've been trying to improve it more based on my heart surgery experience. We give out free nutritional advice and sell a nutritional analysis product.

- I take my meds, turn to help where ever I can find it, I pray a lot and appreciate every day I'm given.

- Though I share the same experience of having a CABG as other patients I was lucky not to have a heart attack. I was never really scared, just happy to know my life was going to be given back to me. Also, I never suffered any depression after surgery because for me it was great to know I could enjoy life again. My first century ride was a challenge but it was one I enjoyed every mile I went.

- I think the sharing on the Facebook group has been incredibly valuable. Also, keeping a month-long Gratitude journal right after my surgery was extremely helpful.

- I think that recovery is just as much mental as the physical.

- Finding the best doctors is important, but in my case it was finding those I can communicate with and have a great rapport with. They have my back and I love the fact that I know they really are there.

- I read and research a lot on new developments that may help with my situation, hoping not to have another heart attack.

- Although the road to recovery might be long & sometimes hard - we're all warriors & we'll overcome our adversities. We just have to keep that end result of achievement in mind and we'll get there.

- When you drop off the social map late after a heart attack, you lose friends and people who haven't got time for the unwell.

Support groups are a godsend.

- The entire process made me keenly aware of mortality. I'm glad to be alive. Life is good and people are a blessing.

- Asking for help is a strength; not a weakness.

- This heart disease hit me and my family like a Mack truck. We didn't see it coming. I'm still scared it will take me away swiftly so I don't leave things un-said, or situations not completed. My husband kisses me every morning and every night. My kids tell me they love me even when they don't :-). It has changed our lives for the better. I sit here writing this with my heart monitor on and a happy full heart to go with it. It may have been a blessing.

- My first cardiac rehab program really brought me back to life. I credit that staff! Finding the right doc who listens was very important. My first cardiologist was a d$ck. Blew off my concerns. Second cardiologist cares and addresses all of my issues. I never feel like I'm bothering her or asking dumb questions. She also showed me my echo. That helped me really understand the damage that had been done.

- I was totally unaware of the process for recovery for bypass surgery, because no one close to me had had it. There have been many things that concerned and scared me, and I there were different answers to my concerns, depending on who I talked to. I wanted a definite answer about how long the recovery process was expected to take, and got answers that extended from 6 months to never. Apparently, each person is different. It has been 12 months now, and I still have little nerve pings in my chest and my sternum area is sore to touch. My left shoulder is still weaker than the right, although I have been using weights twice a week for six months to strengthen it. I still get tired and need to rest in the middle of the day. I doubt that I will get any better from this point on, given my age, but I am doing everything I can to stay active and as fit as I can be.

- Faith played a major role in me being able to handle and stay positive throughout this event. It turned out to be a blessing in many ways as I shared my story and inspired others to get help before potential tragedy struck.

- No matter how bad things seem, live your life doing the best you can with what you have. Living is always better then dying.

- It is through the grace of God I am alive. Yes, it is frustrating to deal with a permanent disability, especially as severe as mine. I was a healthy, active, and busy wife and mother of two when this happened. But through it all, I am healthy, happy, and alive and with my loving family. I am blessed.

About the Author

Word of mouth is crucial for any author to succeed. If you enjoyed this book, please consider leaving a review at Amazon even if it's only a line of two; it would make all the difference and would be very much appreciated.

You can also follow him on Twitter, get in touch on Facebook or through Google+. Lastly, you can always send him an email: eric@booksbyeric.com

Eric Douglas spent his childhood Sunday nights watching "The Undersea World of Jacques Cousteau" and dreamed of diving alongside the Captain. He became a diver, and then a dive instructor, meeting his goals and pursuing a life of adventure and travel.

Through his fictional works, Eric take readers on adventures of their own. His stories have everything thriller junkies crave; action, adventure and intrigue, set against a backdrop beautiful locations, the ocean and the environment, and scuba diving. The fast-paced stories are exciting, but Eric also hopes to inspire future generations of explorers and adventurers like Cousteau did for him.

After completing a program at the Center for Documentary Studies at Duke University, Eric jumped into documentary work, creating nonfiction works on lobster divers, war veterans, and cancer survivors.

Visit his website at: www.booksbyeric.com.

Non-fiction

- Dive-abled: The Leo Morales Story
- Heart Survivor: Recovery After Heart Surgery
- Capturing Memories: How to Record Oral Histories
- Keep on, Keepin' on: A Breast Cancer Survivor Story
- Common Valor: Companion to the multimedia documentary West Virginia Voices of War
- Russia: The New Age
- Scuba Diving Safety

Other books:
River Town

Mike Scott Adventures

- Cayman Cowboys
- Flooding Hollywood
- Guardians' Keep
- Wreck of the Huron
- Heart of the Maya
- Return to Cayman: Paradise Held Hostage
- Oil and Water
- Turks and Chaos: Hostile Waters

Children's Books

Sea Turtle Rescue and Other Stories

Withrow Key Short Stories

- Tales from Withrow Key: Eight Thriller Short Stories from the Florida Keys
- Lyin' Fish

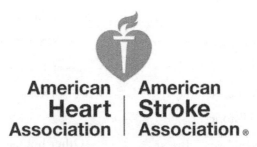

About the American Heart Association

The American Heart Association is devoted to saving people from heart disease and stroke – two of the leading causes of death in the world. We team with millions of volunteers to fund innovative research, fight for stronger public health policies, and provide lifesaving tools and information to prevent and treat these diseases. The Dallas-based association is one of the world's oldest and largest voluntary organizations dedicated to fighting heart disease and stroke. To learn more or to get involved, visit www.heart.org or follow us on Facebook and Twitter.

References

1. Mark S. Link, Lauren C. Berkow, Peter J. Kudenchuk, Henry R. Halperin, Erik P. Hess, Vivek K. Moitra, Robert W. Neumar, Brian J. O'Neil, James H. Paxton, Scott M. Silvers, Roger D. White, Demetris Yannopoulos, Michael W. Donnino, Part 7: Adult Advanced Cardiovascular Life Support, 2015 American Heart Association Guidelines Update for Cardiopulmonary Resuscitation and Emergency Cardiovascular Care; Circulation. 2015;132:S444-S464, Originally published October 14, 2015.

2. Spindler, Helle MSc; Pedersen, Susanne S. PhD, Psychosomatic Medicine: Posttraumatic Stress Disorder in the Wake of Heart Disease: Prevalence, Risk Factors, and Future Research Directions, September/October 2005 - Volume 67 - Issue 5 - pp 715-723.

3. Go AS, Mozaffarian D, Roger VL, Benjamin EJ, Berry JD, Borden WB, Bravata DM, Dai S, Ford ES, Fox CS, Franco S, Fullerton HJ, Gillespie C, Hailpern SM, Heit JA, Howard VJ, Huffman MD, Kissela BM, Kittner SJ, Lackland DT, Lichtman JH, Lisabeth LD, Magid D, Marcus GM, Marelli A, Matchar DB, McGuire DK, Mohler ER, Moy CS, Mussolino ME, Nichol G, Paynter NP, Schreiner PJ, Sorlie PD, Stein J, Turan TN, Virani SS, Wong ND, Woo D, Turner MB; on behalf of the American Heart Association Statistics Committee and Stroke Statistics Subcommittee.Heart disease and stroke statistics--2013 update: a report from the American Heart Association.Circulation.2013;127:e000-e000.

Made in United States
North Haven, CT
29 August 2024

56671501R00068